P9-DUM-950

Sandra S. Lee, PhD
Editor

Traumatic Stress and Its Aftermath: Cultural, Community, and Professional Contexts

Traumatic Stress and Its Aftermath: Cultural, Community, and Professional Contexts has been co-published simultaneously as *Journal of Prevention & Intervention in the Community*, Volume 26, Number 1 2003.

Pre-publication REVIEWS, COMMENTARIES, EVALUATIONS . . .

"A VALUABLE RESOURCE FOR PROFESSIONALS AND STUDENTS. Unlike many of the available volumes on traumatic stress, this book focuses on the larger contextual issues, such as cultural factors and the role of the community. The matters of risk and protective or buffering factors are covered, as is the very important matter of the vicarious traumatization of mental health care providers. HIGHLY RECOMMENDED!"

Ronald F. Levant, EdD, ABPP
Co-Editor,
A New Psychology for Men;
Dean and Professor,
Nova Southeastern University

The Haworth Press, Inc.

Traumatic Stress and Its Aftermath: Cultural, Community, and Professional Contexts

Traumatic Stress and Its Aftermath: Cultural, Community, and Professional Contexts has been co-published simultaneously as *Journal of Prevention & Intervention in the Community*, Volume 26, Number 1 2003.

The *Journal of Prevention & Intervention in the Community*™ Monographic "Separates" (formerly the *Prevention in Human Services* series)*

For information on previous issues of *Prevention in Human Services*, edited by Robert E. Hess, please contact: The Haworth Press, Inc., 10 Alice Street, Binghamton, NY 13904-1580 USA.

Below is a list of "separates," which in serials librarianship means a special issue simultaneously published as a special journal issue or double-issue *and* as a "separate" hardbound monograph. (This is a format which we also call a "DocuSerial.")

"Separates" are published because specialized libraries or professionals may wish to purchase a specific thematic issue by itself in a format which can be separately cataloged and shelved, as opposed to purchasing the journal on an on-going basis. Faculty members may also more easily consider a "separate" for classroom adoption.

"Separates" are carefully classified separately with the major book jobbers so that the journal tie-in can be noted on new book order slips to avoid duplicate purchasing.

You may wish to visit Haworth's website at . . .

http://www.HaworthPress.com

. . . to search our online catalog for complete tables of contents of these separates and related publications.

You may also call 1-800-HAWORTH (outside US/Canada: 607-722-5857), or Fax 1-800-895-0582 (outside US/Canada: 607-771-0012), or e-mail at:

docdelivery@haworthpress.com

Traumatic Stress and Its Aftermath: Cultural, Community, and Professional Contexts, edited by Sandra S. Lee, PhD (Vol. 26, No. 1, 2003). *Explores risk and protective factors for traumatic stress, emphasizing the impact of cumulative/multiple trauma in a variety of populations, including therapists themselves.*

Culture, Peers, and Delinquency, edited by Clifford O'Donnell, PhD (Vol. 25, No. 2, 2003). *"TIMELY . . . . OF VALUE TO BOTH STUDENTS AND PROFESSIONALS. . . . Demonstrates how peers can serve as a pathway to delinquency from a multiethnic perspective. The discussion of ethnic, racial, and gender differences challenges the field to reconsider assessment, treatment, and preventive approaches." (Donald Meichenbaum, PhD, Distinguished Professor Emeritus, University of Waterloo, Ontario, Canada; Research Director, The Melissa Institute for Violence Prevention and the Treatment of Victims of Violence, Miami, Florida)*

Prevention and Intervention Practice in Post-Apartheid South Africa, edited by Vijé Franchi, PhD, and Norman Duncan, PhD, consulting editor (Vol. 25, No.1, 2003). *"Highlights the way in which preventive and curative interventions serve–or do not serve–the ideals of equality, empowerment, and participation. . . . Revolutionizes our way of thinking about and teaching socio-pedagogical action in the context of exclusion." (Dr. Altay A. Manço, Scientific Director, Institute of Research, Training, and Action on Migrations, Belgium)*

Community Interventions to Create Change in Children, edited by Lorna H. London, PhD (Vol. 24, No. 2, 2002). *"Illustrates creative approaches to prevention and intervention with at-risk youth. . . . Describes multiple methods to consider in the design, implementation, and evaluation of programs." (Susan D. McMahon, PhD, Assistant Professor, Department of Psychology, DePaul University)*

Preventing Youth Access to Tobacco, edited by Leonard A. Jason, PhD, and Steven B. Pokorny, PhD (Vol. 24, No. 1, 2002). *"Explores cutting-edge issues in youth access research methodology . . . . Provides a thorough review of the tobacco control literature and detailed analysis of the methodological issues presented by community interventions to increase the effectiveness of tobacco control. . . . Challenges widespread assumptions about the dynamics of youth access programs and the requirements for long-term success." (John A. Gardiner, PhD, LLB, Consultant to the 2000 Surgeon General's Report* Reducing Youth Access to Tobacco *and to the National Cancer Institute's evaluation of the ASSIST program)*

The Transition from Welfare to Work: Processes, Challenges, and Outcomes, edited by Sharon Telleen, PhD, and Judith V. Sayad (Vol. 23, No. 1/2, 2002). *A comprehensive examination of the welfare-to-work initiatives surrounding the major reform of United States welfare legislation in 1996.*

Prevention Issues for Women's Health in the New Millennium, edited by Wendee M. Wechsberg, PhD (Vol. 22, No. 2, 2001). *"Helpful to service providers as well as researchers . . . A useful ancillary textbook for courses addressing women's health issues. Covers a wide range of health issues affecting women." (Sherry Deren, PhD, Director, Center for Drug Use and HIV Research, National Drug Research Institute, New York City)*

Workplace Safety: Individual Differences in Behavior, edited by Alice F. Stuhlmacher, PhD, and Douglas F. Cellar, PhD (Vol. 22, No. 1, 2001). Workplace Safety: Individual Differences in Behavior *examines safety behavior and outlines practical interventions to help increase safety awareness. Individual differences are relevant to a variety of settings, including the workplace, public spaces, and motor vehicles. This book takes a look at ways of defining and measuring safety as well as a variety of individual differences like gender, job knowledge, conscientiousness, self-efficacy, risk avoidance, and stress tolerance that are important in creating safety interventions and improving the selection and training of employees.* Workplace Safety *takes an incisive look at these issues with a unique focus on the way individual differences in people impact safety behavior in the real world.*

People with Disabilities: Empowerment and Community Action, edited by Christopher B. Keys, PhD, and Peter W. Dowrick, PhD (Vol. 21, No. 2, 2001). *"Timely and useful . . . provides valuable lessons and guidance for everyone involved in the disability movement. This book is a must-read for researchers and practitioners interested in disability rights issues!" (Karen M. Ward, EdD, Director, Center for Human Development; Associate Professor, University of Alaska, Anchorage)*

Family Systems/Family Therapy: Applications for Clinical Practice, edited by Joan D. Atwood, PhD (Vol. 21, No. 1, 2001). *Examines family therapy issues in the context of the larger systems of health, law, and education and suggests ways family therapists can effectively use an intersystems approach.*

HIV/AIDS Prevention: Current Issues in Community Practice, edited by Doreen D. Salina, PhD (Vol. 19, No. 1, 2000). *Helps researchers and psychologists explore specific methods of improving HIV/AIDS prevention research.*

Educating Students to Make-a-Difference: Community-Based Service Learning, edited by Joseph R. Ferrari, PhD, and Judith G. Chapman, PhD (Vol. 18, No. 1/2, 1999). *"There is something here for everyone interested in the social psychology of service-learning." (Frank Bernt, PhD, Associate Professor, St. Joseph's University)*

Program Implementation in Preventive Trials, edited by Joseph A. Durlak and Joseph R. Ferrari, PhD (Vol. 17, No. 2, 1998). *"Fills an important gap in preventive research. . . . Highlights an array of important questions related to implementation and demonstrates just how good community-based intervention programs can be when issues related to implementation are taken seriously." (Judy Primavera, PhD, Associate Professor of Psychology, Fairfield University, Fairfield, Connecticut)*

Preventing Drunk Driving, edited by Elsie R. Shore, PhD, and Joseph R. Ferrari, PhD (Vol. 17, No. 1, 1998). *"A must read for anyone interested in reducing the needless injuries and death caused by the drunk driver." (Terrance D. Schiavone, President, National Commission Against Drunk Driving, Washington, DC)*

Manhood Development in Urban African-American Communities, edited by Roderick J. Watts, PhD, and Robert J. Jagers (Vol. 16, No. 1/2, 1998). *"Watts and Jagers provide the much-needed foundational and baseline information and research that begins to philosophically and empirically validate the importance of understanding culture, oppression, and gender when working with males in urban African-American communities." (Paul Hill, Jr., MSW, LISW, ACSW, East End Neighborhood House, Cleveland, Ohio)*

Diversity Within the Homeless Population: Implications for Intervention, edited by Elizabeth M. Smith, PhD, and Joseph R. Ferrari, PhD (Vol. 15, No. 2, 1997). *"Examines why homelessness is increasing, as well as treatment options, case management techniques, and community intervention programs that can be used to prevent homelessness." (American Public Welfare Association)*

Education in Community Psychology: Models for Graduate and Undergraduate Programs, edited by Clifford R. O'Donnell, PhD, and Joseph R. Ferrari, PhD (Vol. 15, No. 1, 1997). *"An invaluable resource for students seeking graduate training in community psychology . . . [and will] also serve faculty who want to improve undergraduate teaching and graduate programs." (Marybeth Shinn, PhD, Professor of Psychology and Coordinator, Community Doctoral Program, New York University, New York, New York)*

Adolescent Health Care: Program Designs and Services, edited by John S. Wodarski, PhD, Marvin D. Feit, PhD, and Joseph R. Ferrari, PhD (Vol. 14, No. 1/2, 1997). *Devoted to helping practitioners address the problems of our adolescents through the use of preventive interventions based on sound empirical data.*

Preventing Illness Among People with Coronary Heart Disease, edited by John D. Piette, PhD, Robert M. Kaplan, PhD, and Joseph R. Ferrari, PhD (Vol. 13, No. 1/2, 1996). *"A useful contribution to the interaction of physical health, mental health, and the behavioral interventions for patients with CHD." (Public Health: The Journal of the Society of Public Health)*

Sexual Assault and Abuse: Sociocultural Context of Prevention, edited by Carolyn F. Swift, PhD* (Vol. 12, No. 2, 1995). *"Delivers a cornucopia for all who are concerned with the primary prevention of these damaging and degrading acts." (George J. McCall, PhD, Professor of Sociology and Public Administration, University of Missouri)*

International Approaches to Prevention in Mental Health and Human Services, edited by Robert E. Hess, PhD, and Wolfgang Stark* (Vol. 12, No. 1, 1995). *Increases knowledge of prevention strategies from around the world.*

Self-Help and Mutual Aid Groups: International and Multicultural Perspectives, edited by Francine Lavoie, PhD, Thomasina Borkman, PhD, and Benjamin Gidron* (Vol. 11, No. 1/2, 1995). *"A helpful orientation and overview, as well as useful data and methodological suggestions." (International Journal of Group Psychotherapy)*

Prevention and School Transitions, edited by Leonard A. Jason, PhD, Karen E. Danner, and Karen S. Kurasaki, MA* (Vol. 10, No. 2, 1994). *"A collection of studies by leading ecological and systems-oriented theorists in the area of school transitions, describing the stressors, personal resources available, and coping strategies among different groups of children and adolescents undergoing school transitions." (Reference & Research Book News)*

Religion and Prevention in Mental Health: Research, Vision, and Action, edited by Kenneth I. Pargament, PhD, Kenneth I. Maton, PhD, and Robert E. Hess, PhD* (Vol. 9, No. 2 & Vol. 10, No. 1, 1992). *"The authors provide an admirable framework for considering the important, yet often overlooked, differences in theological perspectives." (Family Relations)*

Families as Nurturing Systems: Support Across the Life Span, edited by Donald G. Unger, PhD, and Douglas R. Powell, PhD* (Vol. 9, No. 1, 1991). *"A useful book for anyone thinking about alternative ways of delivering a mental health service." (British Journal of Psychiatry)*

Ethical Implications of Primary Prevention, edited by Gloria B. Levin, PhD, and Edison J. Trickett, PhD* (Vol. 8, No. 2, 1991). *"A thoughtful and thought-provoking summary of ethical issues related to intervention programs and community research." (Betty Tableman, MPA, Director, Division. of Prevention Services and Demonstration Projects, Michigan Department of Mental Health, Lansing)*

Career Stress in Changing Times, edited by James Campbell Quick, PhD, MBA, Robert E. Hess, PhD, Jared Hermalin, PhD, and Jonathan D. Quick, MD* (Vol. 8, No. 1, 1990). *"A well-organized book. . . . It deals with planning a career and career changes and the stresses involved." (American Association of Psychiatric Administrators)*

Monographs "Separates" list continued at the back

Traumatic Stress and Its Aftermath: Cultural, Community, and Professional Contexts

Sandra S. Lee, PhD
Editor

Traumatic Stress and Its Aftermath: Cultural, Community, and Professional Contexts has been co-published simultaneously as *Journal of Prevention & Intervention in the Community*, Volume 26, Number 1 2003.

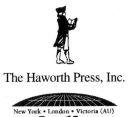

The Haworth Press, Inc.

New York • London • Victoria (AU)
www.HaworthPress.com

Traumatic Stress and Its Aftermath: Cultural, Community, and Professional Contexts has been co-published simultaneously as *Journal of Prevention & Intervention in the Community*™, Volume 26, Number 1 2003.

The Haworth Press, Inc., 10 Alice Street, Binghamton, NY 13904-1580 USA

Cover design by Marylouise Doyle

Traumatic stress and its aftermath : cultural, community, and professional contexts / Sandra S. Lee, editor.
    p. cm.
"Co-published simultaneously as Journal of prevention & intervention in the community, volume 26, number 1, 2003"–T.p. verso.
Includes bibliographical references and index.
    ISBN 0-7890-2181-1 (hard) – ISBN 0-7890-2182-X (soft)
    1. Post-traumatic stress disorder. 2. Stress (Psychology) I. Lee, Sandra S.
RC552.P67.T7556 2003
616.85'21–dc21

2003009783

Indexing, Abstracting & Website/Internet Coverage

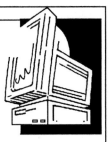

This section provides you with a list of major indexing & abstracting services. That is to say, each service began covering this periodical during the year noted in the right column. Most Websites which are listed below have indicated that they will either post, disseminate, compile, archive, cite or alert their own Website users with research-based content from this work. (This list is as current as the copyright date of this publication.)

Abstracting, Website/Indexing Coverage . . . . Year When Coverage Began

- *Behavioral Medicine Abstracts* **1996**

- *CINAHL (Cumulative Index to Nursing & Allied Health Literature), in print, EBSCO, and Silverplatter, Data-Star, and PaperChase. (Support materials include Subject Heading List, Database Search Guide, and instructional video). <http://www.cinahl.com>* **2003**

- *CNPIEC Reference Guide: Chinese National Directory of Foreign Periodicals* **1996**

- *Educational Research Abstracts (ERA) (online database) <http://www.tandf.co.uk/era>* **2002**

- *EMBASE/Excerpta Medica Secondary Publishing Division <http://www.elsevier.nl>* **1996**

- *e-psyche, LLC <http://www.e-psyche.net>* **2001**

- *Family Index Database <http://www.familyscholar.com>* **2003**

(continued)

(continued)

Special Bibliographic Notes related to special journal issues
(separates) and indexing/abstracting:

- indexing/abstracting services in this list will also cover material in any "separate" that is co-published simultaneously with Haworth's special thematic journal issue or DocuSerial. Indexing/abstracting usually covers material at the article/chapter level.
- monographic co-editions are intended for either non-subscribers or libraries which intend to purchase a second copy for their circulating collections.
- monographic co-editions are reported to all jobbers/wholesalers/approval plans. The source journal is listed as the "series" to assist the prevention of duplicate purchasing in the same manner utilized for books-in-series.
- to facilitate user/access services all indexing/abstracting services are encouraged to utilize the co-indexing entry note indicated at the bottom of the first page of each article/chapter/contribution.
- this is intended to assist a library user of any reference tool (whether print, electronic, online, or CD-ROM) to locate the monographic version if the library has purchased this version but not a subscription to the source journal.
- individual articles/chapters in any Haworth publication are also available through the Haworth Document Delivery Service (HDDS).

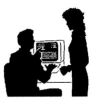

Traumatic Stress and Its Aftermath: Cultural, Community, and Professional Contexts

CONTENTS

ABOUT THE EDITOR

Sandra S. Lee, PhD, is Full Professor and former Chair of the Department of Professional Psychology and Family Therapy at Seton Hall University. In 2002, she served as President of the New Jersey Psychological Association. Dr. Lee is a licensed psychologist and practicing psychotherapist. She has lectured internationally in China and Thailand as well as the United States, and is the recipient of the Award for Distinguished Teaching in Psychology, given jointly by the American Psychological Association and the New Jersey Psychological Association. Her research interests are in the areas of traumatic stress, spirituality, and mind-body interventions.

Introduction:
Traumatic Stress and Its Aftermath

Sandra S. Lee

Seton Hall University

Since September 11, there has been increasing interest in the topic of terrorist incidents and traumatic stress (e.g., Silver, Holman, McIntosh, Poulin, & Gil-Rivas, 2002). This is an important step in the development of the study of traumatic stress, which began in earnest relatively recently, with the study of military combat veterans exposed to wartime stressors. The need to place findings in perspective, and to understand traumatic stress in response to a broad range of traumatic or stressful events, becomes even greater. In addition to terrorist attack and combat, a nonexhaustive list of typical stressors identified in DSM-IV includes childhood sexual abuse, physical assault, sexual assault, robbery, disasters, severe automobile accident, life-threatening illness, or witnessing death or serious injury as a result of violent assault or disaster (see Briere, 1997).

The goal of this special volume is to explore the effects and aftermath of traumatic stress in reaction to life events commonly defined as potentially traumatic, and to examine protective factors which may impact on prevention issues for traumatic stress in the community. An important aspect of this current volume is the varied contexts–group, community and cultural–that are included.

Even before the terrorist attacks of September 11, the prevalence of potentially traumatic stressors in the general population was found to be high, ranging from 39% to 81% of individuals who had experienced at least one major traumatic stressor (Briere, 1997; Courtois, 2002). Prev-

[Haworth co-indexing entry note]: "Introduction: Traumatic Stress and Its Aftermath." Lee, Sandra S. Co-published simultaneously in *Journal of Prevention & Intervention in the Community* (The Haworth Press, Inc.) Vol. 26, No. 1, 2003, pp. 1-4; and: *Traumatic Stress and Its Aftermath: Cultural, Community, and Professional Contexts* (ed: Sandra S. Lee) The Haworth Press, Inc., 2003, pp. 1-4. Single or multiple copies of this article are available for a fee from The Haworth Document Delivery Service [1-800-HAWORTH, 9:00 a.m. - 5:00 p.m. (EST). E-mail address: docdelivery@haworthpress.com].

http://www.haworthpress.com/store/product.asp?sku=J005
10.1300/J005v26n01_01

alence rates vary according to exactly how the stressors are defined and measured. Even so, these rates are alarming, given that many of these individuals have been exposed to multiple traumatic stressors, or may have experienced one event on multiple occasions (e.g., domestic violence or sexual abuse).

Traumatic stress can be severely disruptive, though it does not always result in psychiatric disorder. Traumatic stress may impact an individual, or an entire family, institution, or community. The experience of traumatic stress may be widespread, with a considerable economic as well as human cost. The need for and use of community services as a result of traumatic stress impacting a community may be extensive (Courtois, 2002). The need exists for well-targeted community intervention and prevention programs, to which this special volume can also contribute.

Contemporary developments in the study of traumatic stress are shifting. This volume reflects an emphasis on the study of traumatic stress in normal community, cultural, or college student populations and groups, while other literature has focused on individuals specifically diagnosed with PTSD. The current volume also reflects a shift to the study of cumulative, multiple trauma, and/or lifetime exposure to multiple traumatic experiences, rather than the study of the impact of a single incident of trauma (such as a natural disaster or terrorist incident). This volume in addition emphasizes the search for risk and protective factors, and factors which can buffer the relationship between trauma exposure, and the subsequent distress or aftermath. Finally, the current volume provides the reader with multiple contexts for the study of traumatic stress that reflect cultural and community differences in the populations studied. According to Figley (2002), one of the greatest needs in traumatic stress research is to know more about how groups–social groups, communities, or cultures–are differentially affected by, and recover from, traumatic stress.

Some of the broad questions that guided the development of this volume were: What is the relationship between the experiences of trauma or other stressful life events, and subsequent traumatic stress? What are the protective factors that can buffer or ameliorate the development of traumatic stress in the face of adverse life experiences, trauma, or other stressful events? How do these questions evolve in different cultural or community contexts, and with different populations? What are the implications for interventions for community institutions and mental health workers? The articles in this volume offer a framework for a fuller understanding of these issues, based on a variety of methodologies and measures.

One of the most interesting aspects of the papers in this volume is the variety of settings and populations for which traumatic stress and its aftermath are studied. There are some developmental differences, with the first two articles investigating exposure to violence and traumatic experiences for adolescent girls and also for urban youth. The remaining populations are adults of varying age ranges. But even more interesting are the cultural and community differences reflected in these articles, ranging from adolescent girls involved in armed conflict in Colombia's guerrilla, providing an international context (Hernández and Romero), to a focus on urban African American youth (Yakin and McMahon). Each of the remaining articles provides a different balance of ethnic diversity, and a different setting. Two studies, for example, focus on college student adult populations, to study spirituality and stressful life experiences (Lee and Waters), and psychological characteristics of women who do and do not report a history of child abuse (Lewis et al.). The article by Olson et al. reviews trauma and its aftermath in women in recovery in a community aftercare shelter. The final article focuses on factors affecting vicarious traumatization in a large national sample of female trauma therapists, providing a professional context (Marmaras et al.).

Types of traumatic stressors reviewed in these articles range from a focus on adult and child sexual abuse, to cumulative exposure to stressful life experiences, to exposure to community violence, to forced service in armed conflict, to the indirect exposure of the therapist to the client's trauma. All of the articles, however, address issues related to multiple, repeated, or cumulative exposure to trauma and to stressful life events normally considered traumatic.

With respect to intervention and prevention issues, Olson et al. found that sense of community was high among women in recovery despite high levels of physical and sexual abuse, and the accompanying psychological sequelae. The authors propose a model of shelter aftercare for women in recovery. Hernández and Romero focus on attention to cultural context when designing programs for youth involved in armed conflict. Attachment style was found to be a significant mediating factor for trauma therapists who experience vicarious traumatization as a result of addressing client trauma issues, with secure attachment being associated with less vicarious traumatization (Marmaras et al.). Recommendations are made for supervision and training of therapists who deal with traumatic stress. In the Lewis et al. article, fearful and anxious attachment styles were also higher for women who had been sexually abused as children when compared with those who did not report such abuse. A recommendation is made for special attention to normal populations of women who have been abused as children given the many psychological sequelae of abuse outlined in this article investigating differences in abused and nonabused college students. Yakin and McMahon stress the importance of self esteem as a protective factor for their sample of urban youth exposed to community violence, along with others protective factors that should be addressed in intervention/prevention programs. Lee and Waters found spirituality to be a protective factor for adult college students exposed to lifetime traumatic stressors. A recommendation is made for the inclusion of spirituality, when appropriate, in prevention and intervention responses for traumatic stress.

I am sure you will find this volume to be extremely valuable, and an important step, however small, in our furthered understanding of traumatic stress and its impact on individuals, groups and communities. A greater understanding of the aftermath of traumatic stress, and how our intervention and prevention programs should be targeted, makes this volume a valuable tool for researchers as well as for those designing intervention and prevention programs.

I wish to thank Pam Foley, PhD, and Nina Thomas, PhD, for their careful and thorough review, and insightful comments, for articles in this volume.

REFERENCES

Briere, J. (1997). *The psychological assessment of adult posttraumatic states.* Washington, DC: American Psychological Association.

Courtois, C. (2002). Traumatic stress studies: The need for curricula inclusion. *Journal of Trauma Practice, Vol. 1 (1)*, 33-57.

Figley, C. (2002). Origins of traumatology and prospects for the future, Part 1. *Journal of Trauma Practice, Vol. 1 (1)*, 17-32.

Silver, R., Holman, E., McIntosh, D., Poulin, M., & Gil-Rivas, V. (2002). National longitudinal study of psychological responses to September 11. *Journal of the American Medical Association, Vol. 288*, 1235-1244.

Risk and Resiliency:
A Test of a Theoretical Model
for Urban, African-American Youth

Jeanne A. Yakin
Susan D. McMahon

DePaul University

SUMMARY. This study sought to examine issues of risk and resilience among African-American youth living in low-income, violent neighborhoods. Howard (1996) developed a theoretical model to illustrate the interactions among various risk and protective factors that influence the well-being of African-American adolescents. The purpose of this study was to examine a model based on this work, with a sample consisting of 142 urban African-American 5th-8th grade students, using path analysis. The model was found to be an excellent fit with the data. Findings from this theoretically-based study are discussed within the context of resilience research and implications for intervention. *[Article copies available for a fee from The Haworth Document Delivery Service: 1-800-HAWORTH. E-mail address: <docdelivery@haworthpress.com> Website: <http://www. HaworthPress.com>* © *2003 by The Haworth Press, Inc. All rights reserved.]*

Address correspondence to: Susan D. McMahon, DePaul University, Department of Psychology, 2219 N. Kenmore, Chicago, IL 60614 (E-mail: smcmahon@depaul.edu).

This project was supported by the DePaul University Vincentian Endowment grant (6-26306) and the DePaul Community Mental Health Center.

[Haworth co-indexing entry note]: "Risk and Resiliency: A Test of a Theoretical Model for Urban, African-American Youth." Yakin, Jeanne A., and Susan D. McMahon. Co-published simultaneously in *Journal of Prevention & Intervention in the Community* (The Haworth Press, Inc.) Vol. 26, No. 1, 2003, pp. 5-19; and: *Traumatic Stress and Its Aftermath: Cultural, Community, and Professional Contexts* (ed: Sandra S. Lee) The Haworth Press, Inc., 2003, pp. 5-19. Single or multiple copies of this article are available for a fee from The Haworth Document Delivery Service [1-800-HAWORTH, 9:00 a.m. - 5:00 p.m. (EST). E-mail address: docdelivery@haworthpress.com].

10.1300/J005v26n01_02

KEYWORDS. Resilience, violence exposure, African-American youth

Individuals who experience the same or similar difficult life events often differ significantly in their reactions to those experiences (Reynolds, 1998). Resilience, or the ability to perform well in life despite adversity, appears to at least partially explain the differential life outcomes of youth who have experienced similar circumstances. The perceptions that youth develop in response to a combination of personal and environmental factors comprise a major component in understanding the experiences of African-American adolescents (Lorion & Saltzman, 1993). Howard (1996) proposed a model of risk and resiliency in an effort to fill some of the gaps in the literature regarding African-American adolescents, and to explain differential outcomes among youth exposed to similar environmental factors. Howard (1996) proposed that distal influences (historical, cultural/racial, and socioeconomic factors) affect the proximal influences of personal resources, community supports, and family strengths. These proximal variables, considered the "resilience domains," are hypothesized to influence five variables: risk of victimization, exposure to violence, and a trio of variables that comprise what Howard (1996) terms the "victimization process" (or the consequences of exposure to violence): appraisal of violence, coping, and psychological well-being. The current study uses Howard's (1996) model as the basis for exploring the relationships among some of the aforementioned variables with an African-American adolescent population.[1]

RESILIENCE DOMAINS

The proximal variables assessed were personal resources and community support. Howard (1996) defines personal resources as factors that "enable the child to receive positive reinforcement and develop a success orientation," and in the current study, self-esteem was conceptualized as a personal resource. Self-esteem and community support will each be discussed as they relate to risk of victimization, exposure to violence, psychological well-being, appraisal of violence, and coping.

Self-Esteem

Self-esteem was considered a personal resource, as there is evidence that self-esteem serves as a protective factor for adolescents exposed to many stressors (Dubow & Luster, 1990). Overall, more positive life outcomes have been associated with higher self-esteem, independent of the extent of a child's delinquent and acting out behavior (August, Mac-Donald, Realmuto & Skare, 1996). Further, higher self-concept has been posited to serve as a protective factor preventing a worsening in behavior (Morrison, Robertson, & Harding, 1998). Howard (1996) suggests that higher self-esteem "contributes to a resilience orientation," and that resilience domains will have an impact on what she terms the "victimization process." This is the supposition that one's appraisals of violence and coping abilities influence one's psychological well-being. Research supports the theory that self-esteem may have an impact on how people appraise and cope with events in their lives. Foster and Caplan (1994) compared individuals' perceptions of life events they had experienced with the actual changes that had taken place following these experiences, and found that those with high self-esteem tended to minimize difficulties and report life events to be more positive than they actually were. In relation to coping, some research has shown that individuals with high self-esteem tend to utilize more active problem-solving strategies than those with low self-esteem (Thoits, 1995).

Community Support

Community support is the second proximal resilience domain proposed in Howard's (1996) model. Church involvement, participation in community-related activities, and perceived community support have been identified as important aspects of social support (Holland & Andre, 1987), and these variables were examined as community support in this study. Community support and participation in social activities have been associated with positive behavioral and emotional outcomes. Community involvement has been linked to lower levels of aggression (Rae-Grant, Thomas, Offord & Bovle, 1989) and less exposure to violence. For children at high risk for behavioral difficulties, social support has been found to mediate the development of aggressive response styles (Dubow et al., 1990). A high degree of social support has been associated with interpreting interpersonal conflicts as less threatening, thereby leading to less aggressive responding in nebulous situations. Howard's (1996) model suggests that more community support is associated with less risk of victimization and less exposure to violence.

Social support is also related to more adaptive appraisal and coping styles and better adjustment in areas of high violence. Supportive others can provide feedback regarding appraisal of events and coping strategies (Kaplan, Cassel & Gore, 1977). In addition, supportive adults can teach and model additional coping strategies to help youth gain insight and control over their emotions (Clark, 1993). Social support can be helpful in promoting an individual's ability to work through a trauma by facilitating the expression of one's reactions and lessening the perception of the environment as threatening (Garbarino, Dubrow, Kostelny & Pardo, 1992). Multiple studies have suggested that youth exposed to violence exhibit different emotional and behavioral outcomes depending on the level of social support they experience (e.g., Berman, Kurtines, Silverman, & Serafini, 1996; Hill, Levermore, Twaite, & Jones, 1996). These findings are supportive of Howard's (1996) assertion that higher levels of community support are associated with more adaptive coping and better psychological well-being, even in the face of high levels of exposure to violence.

In sum, there is some literature to support the relation between the two resilience domains evaluated in this study (self-esteem and community support) and the five risk and/or resiliency variables examined (risk of victimization, exposure to violent events, appraisal of violence, psychological well-being, and coping). Next, links between each of the risk and resiliency variables are briefly reviewed.

RISK AND RESILIENCY VARIABLES

Studies have found that exposure to violence is predictive of future levels of aggression in children (i.e., Attar, Guerra, & Tolan, 1994; Fitzpatrick, 1997), as well as psychological problems, such as anxiety disorders, post-traumatic stress disorder (Horowitz, Weine, & Jekel, 1995), and overall distress and nervousness (Martinez & Richters, 1993). Rather than examining risk of victimization, per se (as Howard's model suggests), this study examined aggressive behavior as a risk domain, given its strong connection to exposure to violence. Studies have found that aggression is strongly associated with experiencing and perpetrating victimization (e.g., Schwartz, McFadyen-Ketchum, Dodge, Pettit, & Bates, 1998; Attar et al., 1994; Hill et al., 1996).

A person's appraisal of a situation can lead to anxious or depressive responses (Finlay-Jones & Brown, 1981; Seligman, Abramson, Semmel, & Von-Baeyer, 1980), and the literature suggests that certain styles of appraisal are more adaptive than others. For example, research has found that positive or ambiguous perceptions (Thoits, 1983), controllable perceptions (Taylor & Armor, 1996; Seligman et al., 1980) and perceptions of less violence exposure (Hill & Madhere, 1996), whether accurate or not, are associated with better outcomes. Regarding coping, some research also suggests that active coping strategies, such as problem-solving and seeking assistance from others, are associated with better psychological outcomes (Herman-Stahl & Petersen, 1996; Ebata & Moos, 1995). Other studies suggest that distraction coping may be more effective in particular circumstances, such as when dealing with uncontrollable stressors like exposure to violence (e.g., DeAnda, Baroni, Boskin, Buchwald, Morgan et al., 2000; Compas, Orosan, & Grant, 1993).

There is a need to better understand resilience and both the processes and outcomes that are influenced by personal and environmental factors. Howard's (1996) theoretical model is a step toward understanding the risk and protective factors that African-American youth experience, yet this model has not been tested. The current study seeks to test a model, using Howard's (1996) work as a theoretical lens, with a sample of urban African-American youth exposed to high levels of violence.

METHOD

Research Participants

This study was conducted to examine the risk and protective factors of African-American youth and to examine the effectiveness of two violence prevention programs (McMahon & Washburn, in press; McMahon, Washburn, & Ribordy, 2002). All students in grades six through eight in three Chicago Public Schools were invited to participate in this study. The sample for the current study includes 142 African-American students who completed surveys in the Fall of 1999.[2] Participants ranged in age from 10-15, and included 93 females and 49 males. Each of these schools serves 96-97% low-income students (Chicago Public Schools, 1999).

Procedure

After obtaining University IRB approval, passive parental informed consent and active student assent were gained prior to survey administration. Two graduate students administered the surveys in each classroom, and efforts were made to have at least one African American, and a male and female, in each classroom. The researchers read each question aloud while participants read along. The surveys took approximately one hour to administer.

Measures

Self-Esteem. The first resilience domain of personal resources was assessed by the Rosenberg Self-Esteem Scale (1965). This 10-item scale is the most widely used instrument for measuring global self-esteem (Blascovich & Tomaka, 1991). Rosenberg (1965) identifies global self-esteem as an overall feeling of being a worthwhile person with positive qualities. This measure has been used with people from diverse backgrounds including race, age, and socioeconomic conditions (Wylie, 1989). Estimates of internal consistency for this measure range between .74 and .92 (Shevlin, Bunting, Brendan, & Lewis, 1995), and the Alpha Coefficient for the current study was adequate at .74.

Community Supports. The second resilience domain of community supports was examined through a three-item scale (designed for the current study) that assessed community involvement and perceptions of community support. The first question, "How often do you go to church?," used a four-point scale ranging from never to often. Spiritual support is an important social support utilized in the African-American community (Maton, Teti, Corns, Vieira-Baker, Lavine et al., 1996). The second item asked, "How many days per week do you participate in community-related activities?," with responses ranging from one to seven. Participation in community activities is an important source of support and is positively related to healthy functioning (Rae-Grant et al., 1989). The third item asked, "How supported do you feel by your community?," using a four-point scale ranging from not at all supported to very supported. Coefficient Alpha was .78 for the current sample, suggesting good internal consistency for this population.

Exposure to Violence. The Children's Exposure to Violence Scale (Dahlberg, Toal, & Behrens, 1998; Richters & Martinez, 1990), a 12-item scale, measures the amount of violence that children have personally witnessed, on a four-point scale ranging from never to many times. Self-report of exposure to violence has been found to be the most representative and accurate indication of the amount of violence to which children have been exposed (White, Bruce, Farrell, & Kliewer, 1998). Internal consistency has been found to be .84 with a sample of African-American youth (Richters & Martinez, 1990). In the current study, the Alpha coefficient was .79, suggesting good reliability.

Aggressive Behavior. This risk domain was assessed through the 11-item Aggressive Behavior Scale (Orpinas, Parcel, McAlister, & Frankowski, 1995) that examines the frequency of students' self-reported aggressive behaviors. Students were asked to circle the number of times (from 0 to 6 and above) that they performed a particular aggressive act within the past seven days. This measure has been found to have an internal consistency of .85 with a sample of African-American youth. In the current study, Alpha reliability was high, yielding a coefficient of .88.

Appraisal of Violence. To assess students' perceptions or interpretations of the violence in their neighborhood, a 12-item measure was created for this study. This measure sought to examine three aspects of participants' appraisals of neighborhood violence: the degree of concern the person has about the amount of violence in his or her area, the extent to which the person views the violence as controllable, and the degree to which the person finds the violence predictable. Students responded on a four-point scale ranging from strongly agree to strongly disagree. Appraisal styles characterized by less concern about the violence, more control over the violence, and more predictable violence were considered more adaptive for the purposes of this study, and are represented by lower scores (i.e., Thoits, 1983). This scale had low internal consistency with the current sample with an Alpha Coefficient of .47.

Anxiety and Depression. The anxious/depressed scale (16 items) of the Youth Self-Report (YSR) (Achenbach, Howell, Quay, & Conners, 1991) was used to assess psychological well-being. The YSR is the most standardized and validated measure of adolescent internalizing behaviors (Achenbach et al., 1991; Achenbach, Howell, McConaughy, & Stanger, 1995). Responses range from zero (not true) to two (very true or often true). Internal consistency for this scale with the current sample was high at .85.

Coping. A measure of children's coping mechanisms was obtained with the Children's Coping Strategies Checklist (Ayers, Sandler, West, & Roosa, 1996; Sandler, Tein, & West, 1994). This 54-item scale is a well-validated measure that assesses how often respondents utilize particular coping strategies, from most of the time to never. The measure examines four coping styles including Active, Distraction, Avoidance, and Support-Seeking (Ayers et al., 1996). Distraction strategies were considered an adaptive coping style in the current study, due to the literature suggesting that this style of coping is more adaptive than others when stressors (such as exposure to violence) are uncontrollable. Distraction coping in this measure included physical activities (i.e., playing sports) and distracting actions (i.e., video games or a hobby) to take one's mind off of problematic situations. Responses for the two distraction scales (Physical Release of Emotion and Distracting Actions) were summed to create a total factor score for Distraction Coping, and internal consistency for this factor was acceptable at .69.

RESULTS

Chi-square analyses were conducted to examine any significant gender or age differences within the seven measures. There were no significant gender differences, but there were significant age differences for two scales in the model: the Rosenberg Self-Esteem Scale and the Appraisal of Violence measure. The model was run separately for each age group, and no significant differences in the path coefficients and fit statistics were revealed. The overall means, modes, and standard deviations for each of the scales examined are reported in Table 1.

Path analysis was used to examine the goodness of fit of a theoretical model based on Howard's (1996) work. The Lisrel 8 program (Joreskog & Sorbom, 1999) was used to estimate the parameters for the measurement model. This program estimates the strength of each of the paths specified in the model and provides various fit statistics that allow one to assess its degree of fit. Maximum likelihood was the estimation method used within the statistical program.

To determine the adequacy of the model's fit, the chi-square test, the χ^2/df ratio, the Goodness of Fit Index (GFI), and the Comparative Fit In-

TABLE 1. Descriptive Statistics by Scale

Measure	Scale Range		M	Mode	SD
	Possible	Actual			
Self-Esteem	0-40	3-30	22.38	23.00	4.71
Community Support	0-15	2-13	6.26	5.00	2.75
Aggressive Behavior	0-66	0-66	23.20	5.00	16.54
Exposure to Violence	0-48	1-48	28.95	19.00	6.10
Anxiety/Depression	0-32	0-31	7.00	3.00	5.93
Appraisal of Violence	12-48	17-43	31.47	34.00	4.55
Distraction Coping	13-64	20-59	39.10	41.70	5.85

dex (CFI) (Schumacker & Lomax, 1996) were used. The path-analytic model consisted of seven latent variables: self-esteem, community supports, exposure to violence, aggressive behavior, appraisal of violence, psychological well-being, and coping. Figure 1 illustrates the strength of the pathways (values of $+/-1.96$ are considered significant pathways) and the measurement errors for the model. The Lisrel fit statistics suggest the model is an excellent fit with the data, χ^2 (5, N = 142) = 5.321, p > .05; χ^2/df = 1.06; GFI = .99; CFI = .99.

DISCUSSION

Path analysis was conducted to examine the relationships among various risk and resiliency variables, based on a theoretical model proposed by Howard (1996). This model was an excellent fit with the data and demonstrated the following significant relationships: (1) higher self-esteem was associated with less aggression and less anxiety/depression; (2) more community support was associated with appraisals of violence as more predictable and controllable and with more distraction coping; (3) more exposure to violence was associated with more aggression; (4) more aggression was associated with less predictable and controllable appraisals of violence; and (5) less predictable and controllable appraisals of violence were associated with more anxiety/depression.

These findings suggest that self-esteem did lead to better psychosocial outcomes and was a "resilience domain" for the participants in this study. Community support also appears to be a positive influence, given its association with distraction coping and appraisal of violence. It may be that increased perceptions of support and involvement in community activities lead youth to appraise violence as more predictable and controllable, and this perception may distract them from the violence in their neighborhood. The relation between exposure to violence and aggression is supported by many studies with similar results (e.g., Attar et al., 1994; Farrell & Bruce, 1997). Increased aggressive behavior was associated with appraisals of less control over violence. Aggressive youth, given their high rates of exposure to violence, may perceive their neighborhood as being threatening, which in turn, may lead to more aggressive behavior. Behaving aggressively in a community with high rates of violence may also be an attempt to achieve a feeling of control over the community violence. Finally, appraisals of less control over

FIGURE 1. Path-Analytic Model of Risk and Resiliency for African-American Youth

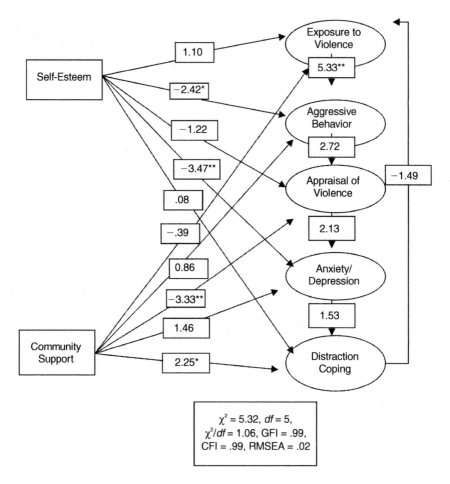

$\chi^2 = 5.32$, $df = 5$,
$\chi^2/df = 1.06$, GFI = .99,
CFI = .99, RMSEA = .02

Note. *$p < .05$ **$p < .01$ (two-tailed tests)

the environment were associated with poorer psychosocial functioning, suggesting that one's view of a situation contributes to one's response. This is consistent with research showing that children's perceptions of the severity of neighborhood violence are more strongly related to their social and emotional functioning than the actual number of violent incidents to which they are exposed (Hill et al., 1996).

Strengths and Limitations

A major strength of this study is that it tested components of a theoretical model developed for African-American youth, an understudied population, using a resiliency framework. Howard (1996) cites the gaps in knowledge regarding resilience in the African-American adolescent population, and this study focuses on understanding the relationships among these variables. Much research has focused on the differences between Caucasian and African-American youth on various factors, but research specifically focused on this population is less common. Flexibility is needed in developing and testing models, and differences within the African-American community should be examined (Luster & McAdoo, 1995). As Gorman-Smith, Tolan, and Henry (1999) asserted, assumptions about other youth, even other African-American youth, may not apply to those who reside in the inner-city. The conditions in these areas may be so severe as to promote behaviors and cognitions adaptive for youth in these circumstances alone.

The limitations of this study include the inability to examine all of the variables in Howard's (1996) original model and measurement issues. First, this study was not able to examine distal influences (cultural, historical, political, racial, and SES variables) and family strengths. Second, risk of victimization may not have been adequately assessed through aggressive behavior. Although risk of victimization is associated with aggression, they are different constructs, and it is unclear to what extent they are related in the population in this study. Third, Howard's (1996) model suggests that many of the variables are inter-related, rather than hierarchical, and the current study did not address the potential dynamic and reciprocal relations among the variables. Fourth, poor reliability was found with the Appraisal of Violence Scale. The inconsistency in responses on this measure may have been due to the three dimensions included within it. It is possible that respondents experience some discrepancy between concern, control, and predictability regarding neighborhood violence. Finally, it should be noted that the inclusion of multiple measures to represent constructs within path analysis is preferable, although not possible in the current study. Because of the lessening of power due to the use of single measures, the GFI may have been inflated.

Future Directions

Considering the early stage of research of some of the variables in the model, more research is needed to examine these constructs and the relationships among them in order to better understand the complexity of the interactions among the variables. The adaptiveness of various strategies for youth exposed to violence also needs to be explored further. Many factors, such as appraisal and coping styles, can affect the outcomes that individuals experience, and these complex processes are not well understood. For example, different individuals may appraise neighborhood violence as significant, but have different reactions to this appraisal (i.e., depression, aggression, avoidance). It has also been suggested that one particular coping strategy cannot be considered adaptive for all people (Lazarus & Folkman, 1984). A general ability to deal constructively with the stressors of life, or maintain high "coping mastery ability," appears to be more predictive of functioning than the particular strategy used (Pearlin, Menaghan, Lieberman, & Mullan, 1981). Exploration of appraisal and coping, in relation to violence, as well as other protective factors such as ethnic identity (i.e., McMahon & Watts, 2002) and family supports, could facilitate the development of preventive interventions.

This study suggests several implications for intervention. Helping youth develop a positive self-view, community supports, and effective coping strategies may serve to counteract the negative influences of exposure to violence. Programs geared toward parents focusing on the effects of exposure to violence, available community resources, and strategies to enhance support for their children may also be helpful. In addition to individual changes that may help children deal with exposure to violence, intervention strategies need to be focused on broader social change. While change on the individual level may prove helpful, the overarching problem of violence in neighborhoods still exists. Public policies focused on improving economic conditions, increasing school funding in low-income areas, and decreasing racial discrimination are necessary to affect change. By taking a broader, more holistic approach focused on the strengths and resiliency of youth, interventions can begin to address these issues.

NOTES

1. In the current study, the distal influences and family strengths proposed by Howard (1996) were not examined. It should be noted that the results from this study may not generalize to individuals whose characteristics on these variables differ from those of the study sample.

2. Some of the sixth grade classes included fifth grade students, so these students were also included in the study. The total sample included 321 students; however, only complete data were used (surveys in which all seven measures used in this study were completed), resulting in a sample of 142 participants. Participants in this study completed surveys at the baseline assessment of a two-year intervention study. Some participants were involved in a pilot intervention the previous academic year.

REFERENCES

Achenbach, T.M., Howell, C.T., McConaughy, S.H., & Stanger, C. (1995). Six-year predictors of problems in a national sample of children and youth: I. Cross-informant syndromes. *Journal of the American Academy of Child and Adolescent Psychiatry*, 34, 336-347.

Achenbach, T.M., Howell, C.T., Quay, H.C, & Conners, C.K. (1991). National survey of problems and competencies among four- to sixteen-year-olds: Parents' reports for normative and clinical samples. *Monographs for the Society for Research in Child Development*, 56, 225-235.

Attar, B.K., Guerra, N.G., & Tolan, P.H. (1994). Neighborhood disadvantage, stressful life events, and adjustment in urban elementary-school children. *Journal of Clinical Child Psychology*, 23, 391-400.

August, G.J., MacDonald, A.W., Realmuto, G.M., & Skare, S.S. (1996). Hyperactive and aggressive pathways: Effects of demographic, family, and child characteristics on children's adaptive functioning. *Journal of Clinical Child Psychology*, 25, 341-351.

Ayers, T.S., Sandler, I.N., West, S.G., & Roosa, M.W. (1996). A dispositional and situational assessment of children's coping: Testing alternative models of coping. *Journal of Personality*, 64, 923-958.

Berman, S.L., Kurtines, W.M., Silverman, W.K., & Serafini, L.J. (1996). The impact of exposure to crime and violence on urban youth. *American Journal of Orthopsychiatry*, 66, 329-336.

Chicago Public Schools (1999). Department of Research and Evaluation School Information Database. Retrieved February 2, 2002 from http://acct.multi1.cps.k12.il.us/.

Clark, L.F. (1993). Stress and the cognitive-conversational benefits of social interaction. *Journal of Social and Clinical Psychology*, 12, 25-55.

Compas, B.E., Orosan, P.G., & Grant, K.E. (1993). Adolescent stress and coping: Implications for psychopathology during adolescence. *Journal of Adolescence*, 16, 331-349.

Dahlberg, L.L., Toal, S.B., & Behrens, C.B. (1998). *Measuring violence-related attitudes, beliefs, and behaviors among youths: A compendium of assessment tools.* Centers for Disease Control and Prevention, National Center for Injury Prevention and Control, Atlanta, GA.

DeAnda, D., Baroni, S., Boskin, L., Buchwald, L., Morgan, J., Ow, J., Gold, J. S., & Weiss, R. (2000). Stress, stressors and coping among high school students. *Children and Youth Services Review*, 27, 461-463.

Dubow, E.F., & Luster, T. (1990). Adjustment of children born to teenage mothers: The contributions of risk and protective factors. *Journal of Marriage and the Family*, 52, 393-404.

Ebata, A.T., & Moos, R.H. (1995). Personal, situational, and contextual correlates of coping in adolescence. *Journal of Resilient Adolescents*, 4, 99-125.

Farrell, A.D., & Bruce, S.E. (1997). Impact of exposure to community violence on violent behavior and emotional distress among urban adolescents. *Journal of Clinical Child Psychology*, 26, 2-14.

Finlay-Jones, R., & Brown, G.W. (1981). Types of stressful life events and the onset of anxiety and depressive disorders. *Psychological Medicine*, 11, 803-815.

Fitzpatrick, K.M. (1997). Aggression and environmental risk among low-income African-American youth. *Journal of Adolescent Health*, 21, 172-178.

Foster, D.A., & Caplan, R.D. (1994). Cognitive influences on perceived change in social support, motivation, and symptoms of depression. *Applied Cognitive Psychology*, 8, 123-139.

Garbarino, J., Dubrow, N., Kostelny, K., & Pardo, C. (1992). *Children in Danger*. San Francisco: Jossey-Bass.

Gorman-Smith, D., Tolan, P.H. & Henry, D. (1999). The relation of community and family to risk among urban-poor adolescents. In P. Cohen & C. Slomkowski (Eds.), *Historical and geographical influences on psychopathology* (pp. 349-367). NJ: Lawrence Erlbaum Associates.

Herman-Stahl, & Petersen, C. (1996). The protective role of coping and social resources for depressive symptoms among young adolescents. *Journal of Youth and Adolescence*, 25, 733-753.

Hill, H.M., & Madhere, S. (1996). Exposure to community violence and African-American children: A multidimensional model of risks and resources. *Journal of Community Psychology*, 24, 26-43.

Hill, H.M., Levermore, M., Twaite, J., & Jones, L.P. (1996). Exposure to community violence and social support as predictors of anxiety and social and emotional behavior among African-American children. *Journal of Child and Family Studies*, 5, 399-414.

Holland, A., & Andre,T. (1987). Participation in extracurricular activities in secondary school: What is known, what needs to be known? *Review of Educational Resources*, 57, 437-466.

Horowitz, K., Weine, S., & Jekel, J. (1995). PTSD symptoms in urban adolescent girls: Compounded community trauma. *Child and Adolescent Psychiatry*, 34, 1353-1361.

Howard, D.E. (1996). Searching for resilience among African-American youth exposed to community violence: Theoretical issues. *Journal of Adolescent Health*, 18, 254-262.

Kaplan, B.H., Cassel, J.C., & Gore, S. (1977). Social support and health. *Medical Care*, 15, Supplemental: 47-58.

Lazarus, R.S., & Folkman, S. (1984). *Stress, Appraisal and Coping*. New York: Springer.

Lorion, R.P., & Saltzman, W. (1993). Children's exposure to community violence: Following a path from concern to research to action. *Psychiatry*, 56, 55-65.

Luster, T., & McAdoo, H.P. (1995). Factors related to self-esteem among African-American youth: A secondary analysis of the High/Scope Perry Preschool data. *Journal of Research on Adolescence*, 5, 451-467.

Martinez, P., & Richters, J.E. (1993). The NIMH community violence project: Vol. 2. Children's distress symptoms associated with violence exposure. *Psychiatry*, 56, 23-35.

Maton, K.I, Teti, D.M, Corns, K.M, Vieira-Baker, C.C, Lavine, J.R., Gouze, K.R., & Keating, D.P. (1996). Cultural specificity of support sources, correlates and contexts: Three studies of African-American and Caucasian youth. *American Journal of Community Psychology*, 24, 551-587.

McMahon, S.D., & Washburn, J. (in press). Violence Prevention: An Evaluation of Program Effects with Urban African American Youth. *Journal of Primary Prevention.*

McMahon, S.D. Washburn, J. J., & Ribordy, S. C. (2002). Training Clinics and Community Outreach: Integration of Service, Training, and Research. *The Behavior Therapist, 25* (5/6), 122-127.

McMahon, S.D. & Watts, R.J. (2002). Ethnic identity in urban African American youth: Exploring links with self-worth, aggression, and other psychosocial variables. *Journal of Community Psychology,* 30, 411-431.

Morrison, G.M., Robertson, L., & Harding, M. (1998). Resilience factors that support the classroom functioning of acting out and aggressive students. *Psychology in the Schools,* 35, 217-227.

Orpinas, P., Parcel, G.S., McAlister, A. & Frankowski, R. (1995). Violence prevention in middle schools. *Journal of Adolescent Health,* 17, 360-371.

Pearlin, L.I., Menagahn, E.G., Lieberman, M.A., & Mullan, J.T. (1981). The stress process. *Journal of Health and Social Behavior,* 22, 337-356.

Rae-Grant, N., Thomas, H., Offord, D., & Bovle, J. (1989). Risk, protective factors, and the prevalence of behavioral and emotional disorders in children and adolescents. *American Academy of Child Adolescence,* 28, 262-268.

Reynolds, A.J. (1998). Resilience among Black urban youth: Prevalence, intervention effects, and mechanisms of influence. *American Journal of Orthopsychiatry, 68,* 84-100.

Richters, J.E. & Martinez, P. (1990). *Things I have seen and heard: A structured interview for assessing young children's violence exposure.* Rockville, MD: National Institute of Mental Health.

Sandler, I.N., Tein, J., & West, S.G. (1994). Coping stress and the psychological symptoms of children of divorce: A cross-sectional and longitudinal study. *Child Development,* 65, 1744-1763.

Schumacker, R.E. & Lomax, R.G. (1996). *A beginner's guide to structural equation modeling.* Hillsdale, NJ: Lawrence Erlbaum Associates, Inc.

Schwartz, D., McFadyen-Ketchum, S.A., Dodge, K.A., Pettit, G.P., & Bates, J.E. (1998). Peer victimization as a predictor of behavior problems at home and in school. *Development and Psychopathology,* 10, 87-100.

Seligman, M.E., Abramson, L.Y., Semmel, A., & Von-Baeyer, C. (1980). Depressive attributional style. *Journal of Abnormal Psychology,* 88, 242-247.

Shevlin, M.E., Bunting, B.P., Brendan, & Lewis, C.A. (1995). Confirmatory factor analysis of the Rosenberg self-esteem scale. *Psychological Reports,* 76, 707-710.

Taylor, S.E. & Armor, D.A. (1996). Positive illusions and coping with adversity. *Journal of Personality,* 64, 873-898.

Thoits, P.A. (1995). Identity-relevant events and psychological symptoms: A cautionary tale. *Journal of Health and Social Behavior,* 36, 72-82.

Thoits, P.A. (1983). Dimensions of life stress that influence psychological distress: An evaluation and synthesis of the literature. In H. Kaplan (Ed.), *Psychosocial Stress: Trends in Theory and Research* (pp. 33-103). New York: Academic Press.

White, K., Bruce, S.E., Farrell, A.D., & Kliewer, W. (1998). Impact of exposure to community violence on anxiety: A longitudinal study of family social support as a protective factor for urban children. *Journal of Child & Family Studies,* 7, 187-203.

Wylie, R.C. (1989). *Measures of Self-Concept.* Lincoln, NE: U. of Nebraska Press.

Adolescent Girls in Colombia's Guerrilla: An Exploration into Gender and Trauma Dynamics

Pilar Hernández

San Diego State University

Amanda Romero

Quaker International Affairs Representative
American Friends Committee
Bogotá, Colombia

SUMMARY. Armed combat in childhood and adolescence is a form of child abuse and a violation of International Humanitarian Law. This study explores the impact of guerrilla life in adolescent peasant girls coerced to join the Armed Revolutionary Forces of Colombia (FARC). It analyzes their stories within the social context of the ongoing conflict in the country. Seven adolescent peasant girls were interviewed with a semi-structured format and the descriptive data were analyzed using the constant comparison method. Results reflect the ways in which they joined the guerrilla, and the traumatic aspects of gendered-based vio-

---

Address correspondence to: Pilar Hernández, PhD, Department of Counseling and School Psychology, 5500 Campanille Drive, San Diego State University, San Diego, CA 92182-1179 (E-mail: phernand@mail.sdsu.edu).

[Haworth co-indexing entry note]: "Adolescent Girls in Colombia's Guerrilla: An Exploration into Gender and Trauma Dynamics." Hernández, Pilar, and Amanda Romero. Co-published simultaneously in *Journal of Prevention & Intervention in the Community* (The Haworth Press, Inc.) Vol. 26, No. 1, 2003, pp. 21-38; and: *Traumatic Stress and Its Aftermath: Cultural, Community, and Professional Contexts* (ed: Sandra S. Lee) The Haworth Press, Inc., 2003, pp. 21-38. Single or multiple copies of this article are available for a fee from The Haworth Document Delivery Service [1-800-HAWORTH, 9:00 a.m. - 5:00 p.m. (EST). E-mail address: docdelivery@haworthpress.com].

10.1300/J005v26n01_03

lence and combat exposure. An understanding of these traumatic experiences is discussed highlighting the continuum of patriarchal practices that make girls specific targets of sexual exploitation. Implications for rehabilitation programs are discussed. *[Article copies available for a fee from The Haworth Document Delivery Service: 1-800-HAWORTH. E-mail address: <docdelivery@haworthpress.com> Website: <http://www.HaworthPress. com> © 2003 by The Haworth Press, Inc. All rights reserved.]*

KEYWORDS. Trauma, war, gender

According to UNICEF (2002) the recruitment of children in armed conflicts currently involves about 300,000 children worldwide. Because they are easily manipulated, children are used as fighters, servants and sex slaves in armed conflicts. Many children join guerrilla groups in order to escape familial abuse and others see it as the only viable option in conditions of poverty. The Optional Protocol to the Convention on the Rights of the Child on the Involvement of Children in Armed Conflict (2002) outlaws the direct involvement of children under age 18 in hostilities and bans compulsory recruitment by governments and non-governmental forces below that age. Child recruitment for combat is one of the many violations against International Humanitarian Law by the FARC (Armed Revolutionary Forces of Colombia) and the paramilitary groups. These left and right wing groups are currently fighting to control the country. According to the US Department of State (2000, p. 7), the Colombian government estimates that these groups recruited approximately 6,000 children. The report states that:

> The Roman Catholic Church reported that the FARC lured or forced hundreds of children into its ranks. It engaged in similar practices in other areas under its control. For example, according to press reports, in June the FARC recruited at least 37 youths, including minors, in the municipality of Puerto Rico in southern Meta department. According to one NGO, in Putumayo the FARC instigated compulsory service of males between the ages of 13 and 15 and was recruiting in high schools. Once recruited, child guerrillas are virtual prisoners of their commanders and subject to various forms of abuse. Sexual abuse of girls is a particular problem. Some 57 child guerrillas were captured or deserted during the year, and 27 children were killed during FARC-military clashes.

As the war continues to intensify in the country and peace negotiations failed, the FARC has increased its recruitment of children by force and coercion. Once they enter military training, they become prisoners. If they are caught escaping, they will be killed.

Several authors (de Silva, Hobbs & Hanks, 2001; Jolley, 2001; Onyango, 1998) have discussed the traumatic effects of child soldiers in Africa, Sri Lanka, Croatia and Bosnia. These include posttraumatic stress symptoms such as hyperarousal, intrusion and constriction. In addition, combatant life impacts the children's cognitive, affective, physical and moral development. These children are forced to engage in destructive, antisocial behavior, rendering them unable to have a normal, supportive social experience. In addition, posttraumatic symptoms may not be evident soon after conflict ceases, but may appear months or years after its end.

The Graca Machel/United Nations study (1996) on the effects of war on children is a comprehensive study on demographic characteristics, and factors facilitating recruitment and effects of participation in armed conflicts. Mendelsohn and Straker (1999, p. 402), define a child soldier as "anyone under the age of 18 who actively participates in a war situation on behalf of a particular group or ideological position." In their analysis of the Graca Machel/UN study (1996), they state that a majority of child soldiers in South Africa, Northern Ireland and the West Bank and Occupied Territories "appear to initiate their own involvement in situations of political conflict and view themselves as fighting for social justice" (p. 403). Children may play a variety of roles ranging from supportive functions to involvement in active combat. In addition, in societies facing great social unrest, children may experience safety inside armed groups. Military participation may offer a sense of purpose and a structured environment.

A key dimension of the Graca Machel/UN study (1996) addressed gender-distinct effects of armed conflict in girls and women, highlighting specific traumatic experiences as well as the important role that women play in children's and families' lives. According to McKay (1999, p. 383), because of their unequal status in society, women and girls in armed conflicts experience "displacement, loss of home and property, loss or involuntary disappearance of close relatives, poverty and family separation and disintegration, victimization through acts of murder, terrorism, torture, involuntary disappearance, sexual slavery, rape and sexual abuse." Furthermore, girls and women are differentially affected in armed conflicts by becoming imminent targets for sexual exploitation. Sexual violence occurs in multiple settings ranging from communities to military, guerrilla and displaced persons' camps. Girls and adolescents are particularly vulnerable to sexual violence, the spread of sexually transmitted and pediatric diseases and abortions. Therefore, the medical and psychological health effects of armed conflict on this population need to be addressed specifically and at multiple levels.

More recently, the report on Colombia by the UN Special Rapporteur on Violence against Women (2002), confirmed the impact of the conflict on the human rights of women. The present study expands on previous research by increasing our awareness and knowledge on the effects of guerrilla life and combat exposure on adolescent Colombian girls through a qualitative exploration of their stories. In order to locate the participants' stories in context, we offer a brief description of the Colombian context and a view of trauma as a social dynamic. An analysis of the interviews follows and initial recommendations are delineated.

A BRIEF DESCRIPTION
OF THE COLOMBIAN WAR CONTEXT

The history of post-independence Colombia can be seen in terms of a variety of complex and diverse forms of socio-economic and political struggles, which frequently manifested themselves in armed conflicts. Massive killings and retaliations have caused more than 4,000 politically motivated deaths per year in the last decade (ICG, 2002). In addition, the long lasting armed conflict degraded with the involvement of armed parties in drug production, taxation and trafficking. Since 1998 reports of the UN Office of the High Commissioner for Human Rights in Colombia have documented the situation, and reports of UN Special Rapporteurs, Working Groups and other UN agencies and bodies have ratified that Colombia is today under a "Humanitarian Emergency." Similar studies and Recommendations have been produced at the Regional Human Rights System (ICG, 2002).[1]

From a gender perspective, Meertens and Segura (1996) and have studied the multiple dimensions that violence has on women in situations of displacement in rural and urban Colombia. They have conceptualized a process by which women develop survival strategies and transform their identities. Destruction, eviction, displacement, survival and reconstruction characterize this process. They assert that the long-term implications of violence for women in Colombia include continued victimization and their increasing participation in armed groups.

Research on women affected and involved in the war at various levels is scarce. However, there is testimonial literature (Salazar, 1993; Lara, 2000) on women who were or have been involved in the Colombian civil war as members of armed groups, as displaced or as indirectly affected as mothers of members of armed groups. These testimonials reflect women's struggle with poverty, inequality, and the effects of decades of violence that have trickled down from one generation to the next. However, no studies have looked at the experiences of girls involved in the armed conflict.

WAR AND THE TRAUMA EXPERIENCE

The concept extreme traumatization addresses a context-based understanding of traumatic experiences, as embedded in the personal and the collective experiences under conditions of war (Becker, 1995). This definition of extreme traumatization frames best an understanding of trauma dynamics in the Colombian war.

This definition contains both individual and socio-political processes, and presenting issues are seen as a consequence of political repression and structural violence. Because of the nature of the present study, the authors used Becker's definition to understand the kidnapped girls' trauma dynamics. Previous studies (Castano, 1994) have already pointed at the need to use expanded definitions of trauma rather than symptom-based definitions.

Studies (Barbarin, Richeter & deWet, 2001; Angel, Hjern & Ingleby, 2001) on the effects of exposure to violence in recent conflicts shed light on the impact of war on children. Angel et al. (2001, p. 5) studied 99 school-age Bosnian refugee children in Sweden. They cautioned that "there is no one-to-one relationship between the experience of organized violence and the occurrence of psychological problems." In their view, supporting research suggests that several issues must be taken into account: the heterogeneity of war stressors and psychological sequelae, the children's characteristics, the influence of the immediate social environment, and the effects of social, historical and political factors. They found that symptoms consistent with PTSD were widespread in their sample and that along with depressive symptoms they could be related to the experience of violent events. Overall, children showed low frequencies of mental health problems and high resilience. However, in a South African context, Barbarin et al. (2001) studied the effects of exposure to direct and vicarious political, family and community violence on 625 six-year-old Black children. Their findings supported previous data indicating a serious negative impact in psychological and academic functioning. Both direct and vicarious violence had an impact in the domains of attention, aggression and anxiety-depression. The present study focuses on the specific effects of forced recruitment into the guerrilla on adolescent girls.

METHOD

This qualitative, exploratory case study was guided by grounded and feminist theory (Lincoln & Guba, 1985; Rubin, 1991). Through inductive analysis, it seeks an in-depth understanding of the participants' comprehension of their lives to gain insight into their social world.

Selection of Participants

Seven adolescent girls from peasant backgrounds, who had been combatants in the FARC between the ages of 13 and 17, were interviewed by four trained interviewers in two Colombian cities. The participants were located through informal contacts with three private institutions that have contracts with the Colombian Family Welfare Institute (ICBF for its Spanish acronym) and the Presidential Programme for Demobilization and Reintegration, and were invited to participate voluntarily. A fee was offered as an incentive. All girls invited to participate accepted. They were selected on the basis of their having had combat exposure in the guerrilla. Their length of time in the guerrilla ranged from one month to 2 and one half years. All but one were involved in one or more sexual relationships by older guerrilla men, one was raped upon arrival to the camp, two had forced abortions, four were engaged in heavy forced labor as punishment, and four had histories of prior child emotional and physical abuse at home.

Procedure

Data were collected through semi-structured, in-depth interviews with each participant, and each interview lasted two to two and a half hours. While specific questions were prepared in advance, the interviewers maintained flexibility to pursue material deemed valuable to the participants. Interviews were audio-taped with permission and transcribed. All participants' names were changed to protect anonymity.

In the first stage of inductive analysis data were sorted and categorized into codes to separate, compile and organize descriptive data (Patton, 1990). This process was facilitated by the software program NUDIST (1993). The researchers used a method of constant comparison, in which the interview transcripts were compared and contrasted to identify recurrent phrases and themes in the data. A consultant reviewed both the initial and later stages of data analysis to add dependability to the study (Lincoln & Guba, 1985).

RESULTS

Theme analysis of the participants' stories is organized as follows: explanations for joining the guerrilla, effects of patriarchy in the girls' lives, sexual division of labor, contraception and abortion, and combat exposure. Interview excerpts were selected to illustrate each theme.[2]

Explanations for Joining the Guerrilla

Children raised in Colombian poor rural communities learn early in life to help their parents with chores in and outside the home. Work is part of their daily life even when they attend school. The girls interviewed complained about having to forcibly help their parents in agricultural, domestic or cattle raising related tasks. They lacked social spaces for playing and for learning through play at home and at school. Their family and community life lacked developmentally appropriate stimulation. This is not an uncommon experience in these communities. Children's work in these poor communities is part of the family's survival.

The most common reasons cited to join the guerrilla were boredom, a desire to wear a uniform and admiration for guerrilla fighters. Boredom was related to a lack of activities stimulating their cognitive and emotional development. Since their parents were raised in similarly deprived environments, they do not have a model to be guided by. In addition, most of the girls experienced a home environment that included domestic violence or abandonment by one of their parents. Traumatic experiences due to physical and emotional abuse at home and loss seem to have been a "normative" developmental unrest for these girls. The interviews illustrate a lack of caring and supporting family environments. Although most of them had at least one supportive adult in their lives, they did not have the spaces and possibilities to grow up as children. In such emotionally deprived environments, the guerrilla life is seen as a better and, possibly only way for change. Young guerrilleros and guerrilleras become role models for the only perceived avenue for a better future within a peer's group. Therefore, these young girls joined the guerrilla out of curiosity, admiration, and a desire to wear a uniform and learn to use weapons. In addition, the state has failed to be present in these communities. The lack of a justice system that works, community health and education services and employment, as well as instances of harassment has opened a space for the guerrillas to make a difference in their lives. Their sympathy for the guerrilla is based on beliefs against the military or their communities' negative experiences with the official Armed Forces.

The Effects of Patriarchy on the Girls' Lives

The interviews illustrate both continuity and disruption of the patriarchal cultural context in which these adolescent girls were raised. On the one hand, the guerrilla experience fits with the patriarchal norms prevailing in Colombia in general and in rural Colombian settings specifically. On the other hand, joining the guerrilla breaks with some of the oppressive practices to which girls are subjected at home (i.e., physical abuse from parents). Therefore, while these adolescent girls talked about ways in which the guerrilla experience offered affirmation and possibilities to make choices, their own patriarchal upbringing made a "good fit" for them to adapt to intimate relationships which can be seen as exploitative sexual relationships from the outside. For example, Carla (age 17) describes violence at home and explains that her mother is responsible for the children's upbringing and that her father, as head of the household, represents authority and good judgment.[3]

> What were reasons for your being mistreated at home?
> Because sometimes my siblings do not obey my father, then, my father says that it is my mother's fault, that my mother did not educate them well.
> Did not educate them . . . ?
> That she did not teach them to obey my father. My mother. . . feels bad because my father is the head of the household . . . The father is the one who should teach the children, not the mother. The mother should contribute, advise the children, but he should be responsible for educating the children. The father is the head of the family that is . . . the most intelligent.

Carla grew up in poverty and stated that as a young girl she wanted to help her parents financially. The community was familiar with the guerrilla passing by and staying in the town. At age 14, she remembered having conversations with guerrilla men about her life and her family's needs. She dreamed of wearing a uniform and leaving home to travel to other places. At age 17 she asked one of the guerrilla men she knew to help her join the group. Soon after joining, a commander, a man in his thirties, became her boyfriend. The following excerpts describe the relationship:

> My boyfriend was a commander.
> Did you have special status because of that?
> No, it was the same for everybody.
> How did your peers relate to you given that you were his girlfriend?
> Well, they did not say anything because they respected me. If he knew anything or if he got annoyed at them, he reprimanded them. They have to respect the commander's girlfriend.
> How was your relationship with your boyfriend?
> Good. He used to tell me that he loved me, that I should never betray him and that I should behave properly.
> Betray with whom?
> With other friends and that I should never escape or leave the guerrilla. That if I had joined, it was because I liked it, that leaving was a mistake.
> What did you do with him?
> We spent a lot of time together, we talked and played . . . he had spent 12 years in the guerrilla, he liked it. I sometimes told him that I was bored there and that I regretted my choice. He said that he did not understand why and that he did not get bored, and that I did not have my parents punishing me anymore.

Susan (age 15), who suffered severe emotional and physical abuse at home, stated that she was advised by other women to choose an older man who could protect her. A 30-year-old man whom she felt was like a father courted Susan:

> He knew that I was still a girl, he told me not to fear him, that he wouldn't abuse me, that he wanted me to be his woman, and since men and women gave us advice, they said that it was better, that I shouldn't pay attention to a younger man, but look up to a man

with more experience so he could help me, then I accepted him. Later, he was my husband, but he was like a father, he used to give me lots of advice and I trusted him with my family issues.

These girls were raised in family environments where men are authority figures who exercise power over them both by force and by seduction. A male figure may be someone to fear–like their fathers–or someone to be protected by–like their lovers. Therefore, when they entered the guerrilla, older men seduced them and they seek their protection. Their submission was both structural and ideological. This kind of continuity between their families' and the guerrilla's social order, illustrates a fit by which they continue to adapt to the patriarchal norms imposed by the guerrilla.

At the same time, the guerrilla's social environment set community rules that may prevent some forms of abuse, and therefore, broke with previous forms of domination. For example, physical and sexual violence toward women is forbidden. Men and women/girls must have permission to carry on a relationship. The girls stated that they were told that they could decide whether to have a relationship with a man and fear no retaliation. This was experienced as a form of affirmation by all of them, except Carolina (age 13).

For example, Sabrina (age 16) escaped her family's physical and emotional abuse by living with a man who also became abusive. The guerrilla, as an organization, forbid the forms of abuse that she previously experienced and affirmed that she did not deserve to be abused through messages by people in the community. Most of the girls, who experienced physical and emotional abuse at home, experienced these guerrilla rules as fair and protective. The community setting affirmed their right to choose whom they wanted to be with, as well as a kind of "respect" that they did not have before. The meaning of "respect" for women in this context protects them from physical abuse. The girls discussed how older women told them to affirm their being respected by not engaging in sexual relationships in a promiscuous manner. Thus, their rights seem to be very tied to their sexual behavior.

Sexual Division of Labor

These girls were raised within family and community environments in which the sexual division of labor was clearly delineated. In these communities, girls are assigned domestic tasks early on in life to help their mothers at home. Domestic work is devalued, and sometimes not considered a job. Elizabeth described this family environment as follows:

> Women had tasks at home, lighter than men's. For example, men used to farm the land and milk the cows. This is their work because they support the family. Women do tasks at home . . . cooking and taking lunch for them. Men don't do these jobs because they say that they work too hard and so on and then one just does the work. They think that what we do is not work, that one does not do anything as a person . . . and one learns that and just does the work at home. That is the custom.

The guerrilla life breaks with these norms stating that "women and men are alike in all respects." Thus, both women and men have to do all kinds of chores for their community. Girls are given both domestic (i.e., cooking) and military tasks regardless of their age. Military tasks involve training, combating and killing others, as well as education to the community. Although girls may initially experience this form of equality as fair, most of them stated that life in the guerrilla was very harsh. They described how military tasks became very tiresome and reinforced their desire to leave.

Since these girls have no awareness regarding their rights as children and their needs as girls, it is important to question ideas about inequality in their home communities and about "equality" in the guerrilla. Both approaches to a gendered division of labor are oppressive to women and girls. However, it is important to rescue the small ways in which the guerrilla experience made a difference: They learned that both men and women can collaborate around domestic tasks.

Control Over the Girls' Bodies

Overall these adolescents talked about having been told at home about their menstruation as a biological event in their lives by a family member. However, none of them were educated about the meaning of this event with regard to their sexual development. In this social environment it is common to assume that a girl's first menstruation is only a marker for their being able to bear children. Families and communities remain silent about sexuality and fear a girl's pregnancy. This fear is then translated into reinforcing the need to keep their virginity and to see men and boys as a sexual threat. Adults and older siblings do not allow them to have boyfriends and may resort to violence to prevent a relationship. In this regard, Ann's story (age 15) is a poignant one. She explained how gossip in town about her having had sexual relationships with a boyfriend became a public issue. Before joining the guerrilla, her family, the school, the whole community and the guerrilla forced her to prove her virginity by taking her for several medical examinations. Her respectability as well as her family's respectability became a public issue. Thus, she had to suffer physical and emotional punishment, before proving to the town that she was still a virgin. Because families had strong links to the guerrilla, she was forced to go through medical checkups to please each group that she was not lying. In the end, she and her boyfriend were forbidden by the guerrilla to continue their relationship. Sometime later, Ann told a young man that she wanted to join the guerrilla. She stated that she wanted to overcome the humiliation by proving to her family and the town that she could be a guerrilla.

Within the guerrilla, community rules affirm their choice of partner by publicly approving their relationships. All members have to ask their superior for permission to have a relationship, thus they can begin and end relationships openly. They do not have to hide, as they had to do before leaving home.

However, sexuality is rigidly controlled in the guerrilla life. Contraception is strictly enforced on women only. All girls talked about how women were solely responsible for preventing pregnancies. Prevention of sexually transmitted diseases was ignored. According to the girls' account they were told that "men propose and women decide." All girls stated that the guerrilla would force them to have an abortion in case of pregnancy. For example, Sonia (age 14) talked about how she and other girls were forced to have an abortion:

> I got pregnant and they did not allow me to have the baby. They took us to the town where we spent about 5 to 6 months. We were 4. They took us in a car to another camp. At night they gave us pills, and administered us some injections, and then we fell asleep. The next day I felt sick. I was very sick for about 2 months, one of the girls almost died . . . she was sent to Bogotá and we did not know if she died. We used to vomit a lot and had stomach pain, we did not eat, and we got very sick and were sent to another town. When we got better, they took us to a doctor and the exams showed that we still had pieces inside and they gave us more medicine. When we recovered, we were taken back to the camp and had to

guard the surroundings. We could not do heavy work. We plead to let us have the babies but they refused. Some women told me to escape but I couldn't because they controlled the whole area.

Sonia and her boyfriend were forbidden to keep the baby and he was transferred to another unit. Sonia, who had already been traumatized in her childhood due to domestic violence, was later victimized as an adolescent. She was both a victim of a forced abortion and a witness of her peers' abortions, illnesses and possible death.

Carolina (age 12) shared that a commander raped her after she had been 8 months in the guerrilla. He continued to harass her and she remained silent until she spoke up and was then transferred to another unit. He did not receive any punishment.

In sum, these adolescent girls may experience some sexual freedom within the guerrilla. They may believe that they have a choice over who, when, when and where they will have intimate relationships. However, control over their bodies in the guerrilla continues to be exercised like it was at home. Women and girls are solely responsible for the use of contraceptives; there is no protection from sexually transmitted diseases; and abortions are enforced if there is a pregnancy. Obviously, they are never prepared for the loss of a boyfriend and a child following an abortion.

Sexuality understood as an overarching frame of identity and development is an area requiring extensive psychological care and education. The social and cultural context within their communities and within the guerrilla life limits these girls' sexuality to their capacity to offer pleasure and bear children.

Combat Exposure

The girls interviewed had different levels of exposure to combat. Although all were trained to use weapons and exposed to war situations, some were not as exposed to heavy combat. Two of them witnessed executions by shooting, and two performed one execution. We chose to discuss this traumatic aspect of guerrilla life through Andrea's case because her story illustrates the sequence and intensity of military training. Andrea joined at age 13 and spent 2 years in the guerrilla. She initially received 5 months in military training. This training included both practice exercises and ideological lectures.

After I joined they trained me and gave me a rifle, then they took me to polygon exercises. After two days, the rifle hit me because I did not hold it hard enough. I felt very scared but later I felt that I was not afraid and could shoot. They taught us how to throw a grenade and how to camouflage. They also showed us films of Simon Bolivar. They say that they follow his ideas.

I felt good because I passed the training, but in combat I felt afraid and screamed . . . I was told to shut up, I screamed too much.

Did you have to shoot?

Yes, I had to . . . I shot like crazy . . . with that fear how could I shoot properly? The second time was not so bad . . . I did not scream but I was afraid. We were like 500. Later, when we got to the camp, we had 8 day training, and then we had a party and drank. That was when I learned to drink.

While in combat, did you see any of your friends die?

Yes, in the first combat two of them died. I felt very bad. The first combat was very hard for me. In another combat, the military captured me in an operation where the guerrilla was outnumbered. Once the commanders realized that too many young men died, they ordered us to leave. They were losing too many people. They were like 200! We were told to get to the ground, and then heavy shooting started. We did not have many bullets. I do not know how I put the bullets in and then we moved, jumped over cords and sticks.

What did you feel?

I did not feel anything, one does not feel, I just continued, I only thought of the objective and how to retrieve. I did not feel, I just jumped and ran.

One behaves without thinking. One does not know what one is doing . . . The commander told me to cover him. I did, but when he jumped and I looked back, he was already hurt. I returned. He told me to take his weapon. I had his and mine as well as the equipment. It was a lot . . . he told me go! Then he died. I told someone else to cover me and as I returned I got hit.

According to the girls, combat training occurs early after joining but exposure may vary depending on the unit location and warfare needs. Because our interviews were not clinical in nature, we did not explore in depth their reactions to killings and executions. Our data are not conclusive regarding the presence of Post Traumatic Stress or other psychopathology. However, we are aware that these girls may develop symptoms over time. It is important to note that Andrea's account suggests how dissociation mechanisms protected her while in the midst of the fight. She denied having experienced symptoms of depression and anxiety while in the guerrilla, but stated that she used to drink heavily.

CONCLUSIONS

Psychologists concerned with research and intervention programs on the psychosocial impact of armed conflict on children must pay close attention to the cultural context in which they are embedded and the differential effects that these experiences have on girls. Girls coerced into the guerrillas face gender-specific violence requiring special attention with regard to their sexual development and relationships with men and women in strongly patriarchal environments. Efforts to develop rehabilitation programs in countries like Colombia should include the following dimensions: the effects of traumatic experiences prior to joining the guerrilla, and while at the guerrilla; sexual development and sexual trauma; education on the larger dynamics of the Colombian conflict and children's rights; and, survival and resilience.

First, these girls' traumatic experiences included physical, emotional and sexual abuse before and while in the guerrilla. Their traumatic experiences can be understood as forms of Extreme Traumatization as there were individual and collective extraordinary events lasting between 6 months and 2 years occurring in a context of confrontation among armed groups (the military, the paramilitary groups and the guerrillas). The guerrilla's kidnapping of children for military purposes aims at their destruction as individuals belonging to a family and a community. These girls cannot go back to their homes because their families are in danger of retaliation for their leaving the group. At the present time they are cut off from their communities and have to continue their lives at foster homes and rehabilitation centers. In addition, they may face stigmatization in the recovery environment. When people know about their past, they face suspicion and mistrust from others. Therefore, trauma specific interventions need to include the treatment of specific trauma related symptoms as well as the multiple losses and stresses of their new environments.

Second, sexuality understood as an overarching frame of identity and development is an area requiring psychological care and education. Since the themes that had most prevalence in the interviews were related to their views on intimate relationships, this is a topic that deserves careful attention in rehabilitation programs. Specific interventions need to address their familial socialization as girls, expectations about marriage, childrearing and occupation, as well as their role in intimate relationships with men. Sexual abuse and abortion experiences need to be addressed as part of this continuum.

Third, a larger understanding of the Colombian conflict may aid them in locating their communities and themselves in the context of the socio-political struggle. Some of the girls openly stated a dislike for the military and a support for the guerrilla. Their sympathy for the guerrilla is based on beliefs against the military or their communities' negative experiences with them. A simplistic view around "the good ones" and "the bad ones" in this conflict would not allow them to take away the guilt and responsibility for a "choice" that they could not make. All of them stated that they made a mistake by joining the guerrilla, and spoke about taking responsibility for their choice as if it was an individual matter. Although they need to take responsibility for their personal choices in the future, a larger and critical understanding of the conflict will help them develop awareness about the ways in which children's choices are limited and the power that adults have over them in this social context.

Finally, a focus on survival and the development of resilience would allow for exploring the ways in which the guerrilla experience supported their personal affirmation with regard to equality in domestic tasks, responsibilities for the community, and choice of partners. The ways in which they survived and learned from the experience will enhance a stronger look at a challenging future. Rehabilitation programs may focus efforts to foster the girls' ability to find supportive relationships outside the family, develop self-regard and recognition of personal power, and a spiritual path. Their reinsertion into educational systems is fundamental to their future survival.

NOTES

1. The reader is referred to various sources on Colombian history to gain further understanding on the context in which this was has evolved. See Franco, S. (1999). *El quinto: No matar*. Bogotá: Tercer Mundo Editores/Universidad Nacional; Molano, A. (1992). Violence and land colonization. In C. Berquist, R. Penaranda and G. Sanchez (Eds.), *Violence in Colombia: The contemporary crisis in historical perspective* (pp. 195-216). Wilmington, DE: Scholarly Resources.

2. All the interviews were conducted in Spanish. Original interview transcripts are available in Spanish.

3. Excerpts translation from Spanish into English was done by the authors as faithfully as possible.

REFERENCES

Angel, B., Hjern, A. & Ingleby, D. (2001). Effects of war and organized violence on children: A study of Bosnian refugees in Sweden. *American Journal of Orthopsychiatry*, 71, p. 4-15.

Barbarin, O.A., Richeter, L. & deWet, T. (2001). Exposure to violence, coping resources, and psychological adjustment of South African children. *American Journal of Orthopsychiatry*, 71, p. 16-25.

Becker, D. (1995). The deficiency of the concept of Post Traumatic Stress Disorder when dealing with victims of human rights violations. In R.J. Kleber, C.R. Figley & B.P.R. Berthold (Eds.), *Beyond trauma: Cultural and societal dynamics* (pp. 99-131). New York: Plenum Press.

Castano, B.L. (1994). *Violencia socio-politica en Colombia: Repercusiones en la salud mental de las victimas* [Socio-political violence in Colombia: Effects in the victims' mental health]. Bogotá: Corporación AVRE.

De Silva, H., Hobbs, C. & Hanks, H. (2001). Conscription of children in armed conflict–a form of child abuse. A study of 19 former child soldiers. *Child Abuse Review*, 10, p. 125-134.

Graca Machel/United Nations study (1996). The impact of armed conflict on children. United Nations.

International Crisis Group. (2002). *Colombia's elusive quest for peace*. Latin America Report No. 1. Bogotá/Brussels: ICG.

Jolley, R.P. (2001). Croatian children's experience of war is not reflected in the size and placement of emotive topics in their drawings. *British Journal of Clinical Psychology*, 40, p. 107-110.

Lara, P. (2000). *Las Mujeres en la Guerra* [Women in war]. Bogotá: Planeta.

Lincoln, Y. & Guba, E. (1985). *Naturalistic inquiry*. CA: Sage.

Mc Kay, S. (1999). The effects of armed conflict on girls and women. *Journal of Peace Psychology*, 4, p. 399-413.

Meertens, D. & Segura, N. (1996). Uprooted lives: Gender, violence and displacement in Colombia. *Singapore Journal of Tropical Geography*, 17, 2, p. 165-178.

Mendelsohn, M. & Straker, G. (1999). Child soldiers: Psychosocial implications of the Graca Machel/UN study. *Journal of Peace Psychology*, 4, p. 399-413.

Onyango, P. (1998). The impact of armed conflict on children. *Child Abuse Review*, 7, p. 219-229.

Patton, M. (1990). *Qualitative evaluation and research methods*. CA: Sage.

Reyes, A. (1994). Territorios de la violencia en Colombia [Territories of violence in Colombia]. In R. Silva (Ed.), *Territorios, regiones, sociedades* [Territories, regions and societies] (pp. 111-122). Bogotá: CEREC.

Richards, T. & Richards, L. (1993). *NUDIST*. Qualitative solutions and research. Melbourne, Australia: La Trobe University.

Rubin, L.B. (1991). *Worlds of pain*. New York: Basic Books.

Salazar, A.J. (1993). *Mujeres de fuego* [Women of fire]. Editorial Colina.

UNICEF. (2002). *Convention on the Rights of the Child on the Involvement of Children in Armed Conflict*. UNICEF.

38   *TRAUMATIC STRESS AND ITS AFTERMATH*

UN Special Rapporteur on Violence against Women (2002). *Informe de la alta comisionada de las Naciones Unidas para los derechos humanos sobre la situacion de los derechos humanos en Colombia.* UN: Author.

US Department of State. (2000). *Colombia Country Report on Human Rights Practices for 2000.* http:/www.state.gov/www/global/humanrights/2000.Report/Colombia. html.

Impact of Stressful Life Experiences and of Spiritual Well-Being on Trauma Symptoms

Sandra S. Lee

Seton Hall University

Catherine Waters

Caldwell College

SUMMARY. Stressful life experiences, trauma symptoms, and spiritual well being were assessed in an adult college student population. Using a regression analysis, results indicated that both stressful life experiences and spirituality were significantly related to the level of trauma symptoms. Approximately 47% of the variance in trauma symptoms was predicted by the model. Spirituality was related to lowered traumatic stress. An additional finding was that trauma symptoms were significantly higher after the September 11 terrorist attacks than before the attacks, when samples from the same population were compared. Results are dis-

---

Address correspondence to: Sandra S. Lee, PhD, Professor, Department of Professional Psychology and Family Therapy, Seton Hall University, South Orange, NJ 07079 (E-mail: leesandr@shu.edu).

The authors wish to thank Abby Sarrett-Cooper and Mary Kelly for their assistance in this project.

[Haworth co-indexing entry note]: "Impact of Stressful Life Experiences and of Spiritual Well-Being on Trauma Symptoms." Lee, Sandra S., and Catherine Waters. Co-published simultaneously in *Journal of Prevention & Intervention in the Community* (The Haworth Press, Inc.) Vol. 26, No. 1, 2003, pp. 39-47; and: *Traumatic Stress and Its Aftermath: Cultural, Community, and Professional Contexts* (ed: Sandra S. Lee) The Haworth Press, Inc., 2003, pp. 39-47. Single or multiple copies of this article are available for a fee from The Haworth Document Delivery Service [1-800-HAWORTH, 9:00 a.m. - 5:00 p.m. (EST). E-mail address: docdelivery@haworthpress.com].

http://www.haworthpress.com/store/product.asp?sku=J005
10.1300/J005v26n01_04

cussed in terms of the moderating effects of spirituality, and current literature on traumatic stress. Recommendations are made for the careful use of spirituality as a resource when addressing traumatic stress in prevention or intervention programs. *[Article copies available for a fee from The Haworth Document Delivery Service: 1-800-HAWORTH. E-mail address: <docdelivery@haworthpress.com> Website: <http://www.HaworthPress. com> © 2003 by The Haworth Press, Inc. All rights reserved.]*

KEYWORDS. Posttraumatic stress, spirituality, stressful life experience

Research has begun to document the association between cumulative exposure to trauma/violence, and symptoms of distress and psychopathology in both adults and children (Figley, 2002; Singer, 1995; Hanson, Kilpatrick, Freedy, & Saunders, 1995; Breslau, Chilcoat, Kessler, & Davis, 1999; Maker, Kemmelmeier, & Peterson, 1998).

Singer (1995) examined the association between exposure to violence and trauma symptoms in large sample of adolescents in high school. Using multiple regression analyses, he found that violence exposure explained a significant portion of variance (about 27%) in trauma symptoms. Edelson (1999) investigated experiences of children who witness domestic violence, and found a range of emotional, behavioral, and cognitive problems. Some of the children demonstrated strong coping abilities. Further research on protective factors for individuals exposed to violence was encouraged.

Exposure to cumulative lifetime sexual abuse stressors events has been found to have an impact on symptoms of distress (Follette, Polusny, Bechtle, & Naugle, and 1996). In a study of the impact of civil disturbances in Los Angeles on residents, it was found that exposure to the violence was predictive of PTSD symptoms more so for persons who had additional lifetime traumatic events (Hanson, Kilpatrick, Freedy, & Saunders, 1995). King, King, Foy, Keane, and Fairbank (1998) looked at variables promoting resiliency in a sample of male and female Vietnam veterans. They found that trauma history and exposure to other lifetime stressors had a negative impact on resiliency.

The present study examines the role of spirituality as a possible protective factor in the relationship between lifetime traumatic stressors and trauma symptoms in an adult population. The positive relationship between spirituality and positive health/mental health outcomes has been reviewed elsewhere (Miller & Thoresen, 2000; Levin, 2001).

In a study of recovering bulimics, spiritual well-being was examined as an aspect of participation in a 12-step program. Subjects' spiritual well-being correlated positively with healthier psychological adjustments (Williams-Biddulph, 1996). In a related finding, spiritual well-being was significantly correlated with positive mood in a sample of HIV-impacted African American and Latino males (Domanico & Crawford, 2000), and with less drug use and better coping in low income women with HIV (Simoni, Martone, & Kerwin, 2002). A buffering effect was found for religious service attendance in a sample of women veterans with sexual assault experience (Chang, Skinner, & Boehmer, 2001).

What impact will exposure to lifetime trauma stressors and spirituality have on level of trauma symptoms? It was hypothesized that higher levels of stressful life experiences would be associated with higher levels of trauma symptoms; it was also predicted that spiritual well-being and stressful life experiences would predict level of traumatic stress symptoms with spirituality associated with lower levels of traumatic stress.

METHOD

These data were was collected in the months immediately preceding the September 11 terrorist attacks. Subjects were 61 graduate and under-graduate male and female college students between the ages of 17 and 55. Subjects received packets containing a demographic data form, and the three self report scales used in the present study. An informed consent form was distributed and returned separately. Instruments were distributed by class professors during class periods. The completion of all instruments typically took about 20 minutes.

Stressful life experiences were measured by the Life Events Questionnaire-Short Form (Pearlman, 1996). This self-report questionnaire (LEQ) measures types of traumatic or stressful events. Sample questions are: "Exposed to life-threatening illness" and "Experienced a natural or human-induced disaster." There are 19 possible life events, including "Other trauma." Subjects may reply with "Yes," "Not Sure," or "No." For purposes of the present study, only the "Yes" responses were counted.

Spirituality was measured by the Spiritual Well-Being Scale (Paloutzian & Ellis, 1982). This 20 item self-report questionnaire yields a measure of spiritual quality of life. The Spiritual Well-Being Scale also yields 2 subscale scores (10 items each) for a Religious Dimension and for Existential Well-Being. The Religious Dimension is defined as the individual's relationship with God. The Existential Well-Being Score is descriptive of the individual's satisfaction, meaning, and purpose in life. The Spiritual Well-Being Scale is scored with a Likert type format, ranging from 1 to 6. A higher score represents greater well-being.

Test-retest reliability, internal consistency and validity are adequate. Test re-test reliability coefficients across 4 studies with 1-10 weeks between testings are: .93, .99, .99, and .82. Internal consistency coefficients across 7 samples ranged from .94 to .89 (Bufford, Paloutzian, & Ellison, 1991).

Level of trauma symptoms was measured by the Trauma Symptom Checklist (TSC-40), which has good reliability and predictive validity (Briere & Runtz, 1989). The scale has been used to measure traumatic stress in nonclinical populations (Elliott & Briere, 1992). This 40 item self report instrument measures the level of various symptom clusters found in traumatic stress. The TSC-40 yields a total score as well as 6 subscales: Anxiety, Depression, Dissociation, Sexual Abuse Trauma, Sexual Problems, and Sleep Disturbance. On the TSC-40, symptoms are rated according to frequency of occurrence over the past 2 months on a 4 point scale ranging from 0 ("Never") to 3 ("Often").

Studies using the instrument indicate a reliable measure. Subscale alphas range from .66 to .77, with alphas for the full scale reported to average between .89 and .91. The TSC-40 and its predecessor TSC-33 have predictive validity with reference to a wide variety of traumatic experiences (Elliott & Briere, 1992).

RESULTS

The sample of 61 subjects consisted of 80% female and 20% male students. The majority (56%) were between 20 and 25 years of age, with a Mean age of 25.83 (SD = 9.68). Most of the subjects (77%) were undergraduate students, while 23% were students in graduate level courses. Self reported race/ethnic identity included: African/American, 8%; Asian, 8%; Caucasian/European/American, 57%; Latino/Latina 11%; Other, 8%; Mixed, 10%. Most (82%) were single, 13% were married, and 5% were separated/divorced or widowed.

The Mean score for all subjects on the level of trauma symptoms (TSC) was 17.11 (SD = 8.91). The Mean score for level of spiritual well-being (SWB) was 93.39 (SD = 15.89). The Mean score for stressful life experiences (LEQ) was 4.83. A total of 91.8% of the sample reported experiencing one or more stressful life experiences (Range = 0-13). Four to 13 stressful life experiences were reported by 55.7% of the sample.

Table 1 shows the correlations existing among the main variables. The only significant correlation ($r = .633$; $p = .000$) is between stressful life experiences and level of trauma symptoms (TSC), such that more experiences of trauma are associated with higher levels of trauma symptoms. The first hypothesis dealt with the predicted relationship between lifetime stressful events and trauma symptoms. Correlations were also examined between stressful life experiences and all of the subscales of the TSC-40. The Pearson correlations for the TSC-40 subscales were: Dissociation, $r = .51$; Depression, $r = .20$; Anxiety, $r = .51$; Sexual Abuse Trauma Index, $r = .57$; Sleep Disorders, $r = .48$; Sexual Problems, $r = .46$. With the exception of Depression, all of the subscale correlations with stressful life experiences were significant at beyond the .01 level.

Results for the second hypothesis were analyzed by means of a simultaneous regression analysis, with level of trauma symptoms (TSC) as the dependent variable, and spiritual well-being (SWB), and stressful life experiences (LEQ) as the independent variables. The $F_{(2,58)}$ was 18.28, which was significant at beyond the .01 level. The R Square was .387, and the Adjusted R Square was .365, indicating that approximately 37% of the variance in level of trauma symptoms was accounted for by the independent variables.

The Table of Coefficients indicated that both stressful life experiences, and spiritual well-being, were significant predictors of the variance in level of trauma symptoms. For stressful life experiences, the Unstandardized Coefficient was 1.54, the Standardized Coefficient

TABLE 1. Pearson Correlations and Significance Levels for Major Variables

	TSC	SWB	Life Exp.	Age
TSC	1.0	−.194	.633**	−.145
		(.069)	(.000)	(.134)
SWB		1.0	.103	.092
			(.216)	(.243)
Life Exp.			1.0	.069
				(.300)
Age				1.0

** Significant at beyond .01 level

Beta was .60 (t = 5.82; p = .00). As number of stressful life experiences increase, level of trauma symptoms increases as well. For spiritual well-being, the Unstandardized Coefficient was −.13, the Standardized Coefficient Beta was −.23 (t = − 2.18; p = .03). As spiritual well-being increases, level of trauma symptoms decreases.

When age is added to the regression equation as an additional independent variable, the Adjusted R Square increases from .37 to .47, suggesting that approximately 47% of the variance in level of trauma symptoms is accounted for by this equation (spiritual well-being, exposure to stressful life experiences, and age). Age is not, however, significant as a predictor variable in this equation (Unstandardized Coefficient is − .15, Standardized Coefficient Beta is − .17; p = .08).

This regression equation using stressful life experiences, level of spirituality, and age as predictor variables was run using each of the 5 subscales of the Trauma Symptom Checklist as the dependent variable. As can be seen in Table 2, the F (3,56) was significant for subscales of Dissociation, Anxiety, Sexual Abuse Trauma Index, Sleep Disorder, and Sexual Problems. The F was not significant for Depression. As indicated in Table 2, the approximate amount of variance in the subscale scores explained by the regression equation varied from 24% to 45% for the significant subscales.

An additional analysis was run comparing the Mean scores of the present sample (N = 61) on the level of trauma symptoms with the Mean scores of an independent sample (N = 125) collected from the same population in the months immediately after the terrorist attacks of September 11, 2001 (Waters & Lee, 2002). The study variables and conditions were identical to those in the present study, where data were

TABLE 2. Regression Equation Results with Subscales of the Trauma Symptom Checklist-40

	F	Sig.	R Square	Adj. R Sq
Dissociation	11.70	.00	.39	.35
Depression	2.17	.10	.10	.06
Anxiety	9.67	.00	.34	.31
Sexual Abuse	15.45	.00	.67	.45
Sleep Disorder	7.13	.00	.28	.24
Sexual Problems	10.43	.00	.36	.32

Note. Predictor variables are: life experiences of trauma/violence, level of spirituality, and age.

collected in the months immediately preceding the September 11 attacks.

Before 9/11/2001, the Mean score on the TSC-40 in the present study was 17.11 (SD = 8.91). After 9/11, the Mean score on the TSC-40 from an independent sample in the same population was 28.69 (SD = 18.06). In the t-test for Equality of Means, the t was -5.85 (df = 184), and this was significant at beyond the .01 level.

DISCUSSION

A noteworthy finding of the present research is the fact that 47% of the variance in trauma symptoms in this adult college student population is explained by the variables of stressful life experiences and spiritual well-being, along with age. The findings suggest that indeed spiritual well being can act as a buffer to traumatic stress associated with cumulative or multiple exposure to traumatic stressors. The current research also supports and adds to past research regarding the strong relationship between cumulative exposure to lifetime stressors, and trauma symptoms.

These findings can be viewed in terms of the broader literature on the positive association between spirituality and health outcomes, now extensively documented (see Levin, 2001; Miller & Thoresen, 2000). The current findings add a piece to this literature suggesting that spirituality can act as a buffer or protective factor in the relationship between lifetime exposure to stressful experiences, and the resulting traumatic stress.

In terms of the clinical and community prevention implications of these findings, therapists and counselors should be aware of the protective effects that can be provided by spirituality in buffering the effects of traumatic stress. This may be especially true for individuals for whom spirituality is already important, and future research would help to clarify this point. In any community or clinical effort to reinforce adaptive coping in response to trauma or violence, spirituality should not be ignored as a possible factor affecting resilience and providing some measure of protection against distress. It is not yet clear to what extent spirituality can or should be introduced as a resource where there is not already a foundation for this. Caution should prevail, and future research can clarify these points.

The prevalence of exposure to lifetime stressors reported by this adult college student population, prior to the events of 9/11, was high–92% reported experiencing at least one of the major lifetime traumatic stressors, and 56% of the sample reported four or more of the stressful experiences. While somewhat higher, these figures are consistent with other surveys of the general population (see Briere, 1997; Courtois, 2002).

The impact of spirituality as a buffering or protective factor in the aftermath of traumatic stress should be explored further in future research, replicating the present study with single incident traumatic experiences, as well as with cumulative stressful life experiences. The search for protective factors in the study of traumatic stress is an important one, and a greater understanding of the role and functioning of spirituality as a protective factor will be a valuable resource.

REFERENCES

Brady, J.L., Guy, J.D., Poelstra, P.L., & Brokaw, B.F. (1999). Vicarious traumatization, spirituality, and the treatment of sexual abuse survivors: A national survey of women psychotherapists. *Professional Psychology: Research and Practice, 30* (4), 386-393.

Breslau, N., Chilcoat, H.C., Kessler, R.C., & Davis, G.C. (1999). Previous exposure to trauma and PTSD effects of subsequent trauma: Results from the Detroit area survey of trauma. *American Journal of Psychiatry, 156* (6), 902.

Briere, J. (1997). *The psychological assessment of adult posttraumatic states.* Washington, DC: American Psychological Association.

Briere, J., & Runtz, M. (1989). The Trauma Symptom Checklist (TSC-33): Early data on a new scale. *Journal of Interpersonal Violence, 4,* 154-163.

Bufford, R.K., Paloutzian, R.F., & Ellison, C.W. (1991). Norms for the Spiritual Well-Being Scale. *Journal of Psychology and Theology, 19* (1), 56-70.

Chang, B., Skinner, K., & Boehmer, U. (2001). Religion and mental health among women veterans with sexual assault experience. *International Journal of Psychiatry in Medicine, Vol. 31(1),* 77-95.

Courtois, C. (2002). Traumatic stress studies: The need for curricula inclusion. *Journal of Trauma Practice, Vol. 1 (1),* 33-57.

Domanico, R., & Crawford, I. (2000). Psychological distress among HIV-impacted African-American and Latino males. *Journal of Prevention & Intervention in the Community, 19*(1), 55-78.

Edelson, J.L. (1999). Children's witnessing of adult domestic violence. *Journal of Interpersonal Violence, 14* (8), 839-870.

Elliott, D. & Briere, J. (1992). Sexual abuse trauma among professional women: Validating the Trauma Symptom Checklist-40 (TSC-40). *Child Abuse & Neglect, 16,* 391-398.

Figley, C. (2002). Origins of traumatology and prospects for the future, Part 1. *Journal of Trauma Practice, Vol. 1 (1),* 17-32.

Follette, V. M., Polusny, M. M., Bechtle, A. E., & Naugle, A.E. (1996). Cumulative trauma: The impact of child sexual abuse, adult sexual assault, and spouse abuse. *Journal of Traumatic Stress, 9*, 25-35.

Hanson, R.S., Kilpatrick, D.G., Freedy, J.R., & Saunders, B.E. (1995). Los Angeles County after the 1992 civil disturbances: Degree of exposure and impact on mental health. *Journal of Consulting and Clinical Psychology, 63*(6), 987-996.

King, D.W., King, L.A., Foy, D.W., Keane, T.M., & Fairbank, J.A. (1998). Posttraumatic stress disorder in a national sample of female and male Vietnam veterans: Risk factors, war-zone stressors, and resilience-recovery variables. *Journal of Abnormal Psychology, 108* (1), 164-170.

Levin, J. (2001). *God, faith, and health: Exploring the spirituality-healing connection.* New York: John Wiley & Sons, Inc.

Maker, A.H., Kemmelmeier, M., & Peterson, C. (1998). Long-term psychological consequences in women of witnessing parental physical conflict and experiencing abuse in childhood. *Journal of Interpersonal Violence, 13* (5), 574-589.

Miller, W. R., & Thoresen, C. E. (2000). Spirituality and health. In W. R. Miller (Ed.), *Integrating spirituality into treatment* (pp. 3-18). Washington, DC: American Psychological Association.

Paloutzian, R.F., & Ellison, D.W. (1982). Loneliness, spiritual well-being and the quality of life. In L.A. Peplau and D. Perlman (Eds.), *Loneliness: A sourcebook of current theory, research & therapy*. NY: Wiley, 224-237.

Pearlman, L.A. (1996). Psychometric review of TSI Life Event Questionnaire (LEQ). In B.H. Stamm (Ed.). *Measurement of stress, trauma, and adaptation*. Lutherville, MD: Sidran Press.

Simoni, J., Martone, M., & Kerwin, J. (2002). Spirituality and psychological adaptation among women with HIV/AIDS: Implications for counseling. *Journal of Counseling Psychology, 49 (2)*, 139-147.

Singer, M. (1995). Adolescents' exposure to violence and associated symptoms of psychological trauma. *Journal of the American Medical Association*, 273(6), 477-482.

Waters, C. & Lee, S. (2002). Pre and post 9/11: Comparison of trauma symptoms, spirituality, and exposure to stressful life experiences. Unpublished paper.

Williams-Biddulph, K. (1996). Spiritual well-being and psychological adjustment in recovering bulimic women. Unpublished doctoral dissertation, Seton Hall University.

Psychological Characteristics of Women Who Do or Do Not Report a History of Sexual Abuse

Robin J. Lewis

Old Dominion University
Virginia Consortium Program in Clinical Psychology

Jessica L. Griffin

Virginia Consortium Program in Clinical Psychology

Barbara A. Winstead
Jennifer A. Morrow

Old Dominion University
Virginia Consortium Program in Clinical Psychology

Courtney P. Schubert

Old Dominion University

SUMMARY. Childhood sexual abuse (CSA) is a prevalent form of violence in our society. The exact number of women sexually abused as

---

Address correspondence to: Robin J. Lewis, Department of Psychology, Old Dominion University, Norfolk, VA 23529-0267 (E-mail: rlewis@odu.edu).

This research is part of Jessica L. Griffin's dissertation at the Virginia Consortium, supervised by Robin J. Lewis.

[Haworth co-indexing entry note]: "Psychological Characteristics of Women Who Do or Do Not Report a History of Sexual Abuse." Lewis, Robin J. et al. Co-published simultaneously in *Journal of Prevention & Intervention in the Community* (The Haworth Press, Inc.) Vol. 26, No. 1, 2003, pp. 49-65; and: *Traumatic Stress and Its Aftermath: Cultural, Community, and Professional Contexts* (ed: Sandra S. Lee) The Haworth Press, Inc., 2003, pp. 49-65. Single or multiple copies of this article are available for a fee from The Haworth Document Delivery Service [1-800-HAWORTH, 9:00 a.m. - 5:00 p.m. (EST). E-mail address: docdelivery@haworthpress.com].

10.1300/J005v26n01_05

children is not known, as the estimated rates vary from 6% to 62%. This study examined the psychological characteristics of women with and without a history of CSA. A nonclinical sample of 255 undergraduate women served as volunteer participants. The variables measured included: Adult Romantic Attachment, Depression, Anxiety, Traumatic Symptoms, Cognitive Distortions, Maladaptive Schemas, and Borderline Personality Features. Women who reported a history of abuse evidenced marked differences from those who did not across a broad spectrum of variables. A majority of CSA survivors did not seek any treatment. These results are discussed relative to prevention and early intervention efforts that are necessary to assist this underserved population. *[Article copies available for a fee from The Haworth Document Delivery Service: 1-800-HAWORTH. E-mail address: <docdelivery@haworthpress.com> Website: <http://www.HaworthPress.com> © 2003 by The Haworth Press, Inc. All rights reserved.]*

KEYWORDS. Sexual abuse, trauma

Childhood sexual abuse (CSA) is a prevalent form of violence in our society. The exact number of women sexually abused as children is not known, as the estimated rates vary from 6% to 62% in society (Finkelhor, Hotaling, Lewis, & Smith, 1990; Meichenbaum, 1995). Some studies have demonstrated that one-third of women and one-sixth of men in our culture have experienced sexual contact with someone substantially older by mid-adolescence (Finkelhor et al., 1990; Wyatt, 1985).

The purpose of this study was to compare the psychological characteristics of women in a nonclinical sample who report a history of CSA to those who do not. If we can specify the differences between these two groups, it will then be possible to develop prevention and early intervention strategies to improve the functioning of these trauma survivors. We also examined the relationship of a history of CSA to seeking professional help.

Childhood sexual abuse is a major risk factor for a multitude of short-term problems as well as difficulties later in life (Finkelhor, 1990; Kendall-Tackett, Williams, & Finkelhor, 1993). Adult survivors of CSA may internalize pain related to their abuse (resulting in affective symptoms such as anxiety and depression) as well as externalize it (producing behavioral problems and interpersonal difficulties). This range of abuse-related internalization and externalization has been documented across race and socioeconomic status (Stein, Golding, Siegel, Burnam, & Sorensen, 1988). Childhood sexual abuse is associated with a four times greater lifetime risk for major depression (e.g., Hall, Sachs, Rayens, & Lutenbacher, 1993; Stein et al., 1988) and up to a five times greater likelihood of an anxiety disorder (Saunders, Villeponteaux, Lipovsky, & Kilpatrick, 1992). Not surprisingly, CSA is associated with a nearly four-fold increased lifetime risk for any psychiatric disorder and with a three-fold risk for substance abuse (Finkelhor & Dziuba-Leatherman, 1994). One specific disorder that has been associated with CSA and other childhood trauma is Borderline Personality Disorder. Trull (2001) found that childhood abuse accounts for unique variance in borderline features that cannot be accounted for by parental psychopathology or personality traits.

The severity of childhood sexual abuse is also related to difficulty in establishing adult interpersonal relationships (Alexander, 1993; Busby, Glenn, Steggell, & Adamson, 1993). Survivors of CSA have fewer friends, decreased satisfaction in their relationships, greater interpersonal discomfort and sensitivity, and more maladaptive interpersonal patterns (Elliott, 1994). Sexual abuse survivors are also more likely to become involved in abusive sexual or romantic relationships and experience revictimization in their adult lives (Sorensen, Siegel, Golding, & Stein, 1991) and one-third grow up to continue a pattern of dysfunctional or abusive parenting (Oliver, 1993).

Childhood sexual abuse has also been shown to result in Post Traumatic Stress Disorder (PTSD) in up to 36% of adult survivors of CSA. For those survivors who experienced penetration, the risk of PTSD appears to be much higher (Saunders et al., 1992). Approximately one-third of female sexual abuse survivors meet diagnostic criteria for Acute Stress Disorder and indicate that interpersonal relationships are the most frequently reported source of acute stress (Koopman, Gore-Felton, & Spiegel, 1997).

Despite the aforementioned negative consequences of CSA, a substantial number of sexually abused children are asymptomatic (e.g., 25-30%; see Finkelhor, 1990 for a review). A recent meta-analysis (Rind, Tromovitch, & Bauserman, 1998) found a weak, albeit statistically significant, correlation between CSA and psychological adjustment. Other researchers, however (e.g., Dallam et al., 2001; Ondersma et al., 2001), have criticized Rind et al.'s methodology and interpretation of findings and suggest a stronger association between CSA and adjustment.

It has been postulated that symptoms tend to fluctuate over time rather than improve in linear fashion (Friedrich & Reams, 1987). Some individuals suffer from severe and chronic symptomatology, some demonstrate moderate and acute symptoms immediately following the trauma, some demonstrate symptoms several years following a trauma following an asymptomatic period (e.g., the "sleeper effect"), while others remain asymptomatic throughout their lives (Finkelhor, 1990; Kendall-Tackett et al., 1993).

The purpose of this research was to compare the psychological characteristics of women who report a history of CSA to those who do not. The nonclinical sample chosen allows us to compare these groups of women without the necessary presence of symptomatology that characterizes clinical samples. This comparison represents an important step in understanding the characteristics of trauma survivors.

We hypothesized that there would be differences between women with a history of CSA and those without such a history. CSA survivors were expected to report more trauma symptoms (e.g., sexual disturbances, sleep disturbances, hypervigilance, etc.), depression, anxiety, and borderline features. We also expected CSA survivors to report more insecure attachment. Finally, we also expected CSA to be related to clinical elevations (i.e., scores above cut-offs that indicate moderate to severe difficulties) in anxiety, depression, and borderline features.

METHOD

Participants

Two hundred fifty-five participants were recruited through the Psychology Department at a mid-sized urban university in the Southeastern United States. Participants received partial course credit in exchange for their participation. Participants were also eligible for a raffle drawing for one of several gift certificates. The mean age of the participants was 21.53 years (SD = 4.01). The mean educational level was 14.29 years (SD = 1.38). Fifty-five percent of the sample were Caucasian, 33% were African American, 6% were Hispanic, 4% were Asian American/Pacific Islander, and 2% reported their race as "other." Sixty-six percent of the participants reported they were in a romantic relationship (including marriage), and 89% were single. Thirty-nine percent of the sample had either been in treatment previously or were in treatment at the time of the study and 7.6% overall were in treatment at the time data were collected.

Materials

Demographic Information Sheet. On the demographic sheet, participants indicated their age, ethnicity, level of education, marital status, and current and past use of mental health services.

Wyatt Sexual History Questionnaire. A modified version of the Wyatt Sexual History Questionnaire (WSHQ; Wyatt, 1985) was used to assess child sexual abuse. The original WSHQ is a 478-item structured interview. Eight questions, targeting touch, exhibitionism, and penetration, were used in written format with the addition of the qualifiers "Before the age of 18" and "Unwanted." Responses to the questions on this measure were used to classify participants into groups based on their experiences with CSA. The original interview format of this measure has established inter-rater reliability (.82 to 1.0) (Wyatt, 1985). A number of other researchers have used an adapted questionnaire version of the measure as we did. Fleming, Mullen, Sibthorpe, Attewell, and Bammer (1998) found that CSA (using their questionnaire version) interacted with several other factors to predict alcohol abuse. Mitchell (1999) used seven items adapted from the Wyatt interview and reported an alpha coefficient of .92. Others using a questionnaire version of the Wyatt found that CSA was associated with negative attitudes toward sexuality, hard-substance use, and more adult victimization (Johnsen & Harlow, 1996).

The Cognitive Distortion Scales. The Cognitive Distortion Scales (CDS; Briere, 2000) measure five types of cognitive symptoms or distortions found among mental health clients and/or those who have experienced interpersonal victimization. Respondents use a 5-point Likert-type scale ranging from 1 (*never*) to 5 (*very often*) to rate how much they have had a particular thought or feeling in the last month. T-scores are created for each of five types of distortions: self-criticism, self-blame, helplessness, hopelessness, and preoccupation with danger. The CDS has good psychometric properties with subscale alphas ranging from .89 to .97 (Briere, 2000). Construct, predictive, and convergent validity were established in both general population and clinical samples. Specifically, construct validity was measured by examining the relationship between CDS scales and suicidality, interpersonal victimization, posttraumatic stress, and depression (Briere, 2000). Internal consistencies of the five subscales in this study ranged from .89 to .95.

The Young Schema Questionnaire–Short Form. The Young Schema Questionnaire (YSQ-SF; Young & Brown, 1994). The YSQ-SF is a 75-item measure that assesses schemas of self in relation to the environment. The measure focuses on "early maladaptive schemas" that are dysfunctional in some significant and recurring manner, and are the result of early problematic interpersonal experiences. The following maladaptive themes in this study were: Disconnection and Rejection, Impaired Autonomy and Performance, Impaired Limits, Other-Directedness, and Overvigilance and Inhibition. The YSQ-SF has been validated on both clinical and nonclinical populations (Schmidt, Joiner, Young, & Telch, 1995). The YSQ-SF is internally consistent with overall alpha levels of .96 for a bulimic sample and .92 for the normative sample and subscale alphas greater than .80 for each group on all subscales (Waller, Meyer, & Ohanian, 2001). The YSQ-SF demonstrates sound discriminative and predictive validities (Waller et al., 2001). Coefficient alphas for the theme scales in this study ranged from .80 to .94.

Experiences in Close Relationships (ECR). Brennan, Clark, and Shaver (1998) created this multi-item measure of adult romantic attachment from a combination of 60 different attachment constructs. This measure provides a common metric for assessing adult romantic attachment styles. Brennan et al. (1998) found two main factors common to all of the attachment measures and constructs: Anxiety and Avoidance. The resulting measure has 36 items (two 18-item scales). Internal consistency was reported to be good with alpha coefficients of .95 for both Anxiety and Avoidance (Brennan et al., 1998). Validity was demonstrated by correlations between the Anxiety scale and scales measuring anxiety and preoccupation with attachment, jealousy, and fear of rejection. The Avoidance scale correlates highly with scales that measure avoidance and discomfort with closeness (Brennan et al., 1998).

The alpha coefficients in this study were .94 for the Avoidance subscale and .93 for the Anxiety subscale. In addition to obtaining scores on the Anxiety and Avoidance subscales, participants can be classified into adult attachment groups: Secure (low anxiety, low avoidance); Fearful (high anxiety, high avoidance); Preoccupied (high anxiety, low avoidance); and Dismissing (low anxiety, high avoidance).

The Beck Depression Inventory. The Beck Depression Inventory–2nd edition (BDI-II; Beck, 1996) is a widely used self-report method for assessing the severity of depression. The BDI-II contains 21 items, each rated from 0 (*not present*) to 3 (*severe*). The BDI has demonstrated good psychometric properties (Beck, Steer, & Brown, 1996). Alpha coefficients were .92 for outpatients and .93 for college students. One-week test-retest reliability was .93. Construct validity was demonstrated by correlating the BDI-II with other measures of anxiety and depression (Beck et al., 1996). The alpha coefficient in this study was .92.

The Beck Anxiety Inventory. The Beck Anxiety Inventory (BAI, Beck, 1990) is a widely used method of assessing anxiety. The BAI contains 21 items, each rated from 0 to 3, representing the level of severity of the symptom of anxiety. The BAI has demonstrated good reliability and validity (Beck, Epstein, Brown, & Steer, 1988). Internal consistency was demonstrated with an alpha coefficient of .92. One-week test-retest reliability was .75. Validity was demonstrated by correlating the BAI with other measures of anxiety. Also, the BAI successfully discriminated those with anxiety disorders from those with depressive disorders (Beck et al., 1988). The alpha coefficient in this study was .90.

The Trauma Symptom Checklist. The Trauma Symptom Checklist (TSC-40; Briere, 1996) is a 40-item self-report Likert-type scale intended for research purposes with answers ranging from 0 (*never*) to 3 (*often*). The TSC measures the traumatic impact of childhood abuse and has six subscales: anxiety, depression, sexual abuse trauma, sexual problems, sleep disturbances, and dissociation. The TSC-40 has good internal consistency with subscale alphas ranging from .66 to .77 and full-scale alphas ranging from .89 to .91 (Briere, 1996). This measure also has good predictive validity regarding childhood sexual victimization (Elliott & Briere, 1992). Alpha coefficients for the subscales in this study ranged from .70 to .83.

The Personality Assessment Inventory–Borderline Features Scale. The Borderline Features scale of the Personality Assessment Inventory (PAI-BOR; Morey, 1991) is a 24-item subscale of the PAI that assesses borderline personality patterns with four six-item subscales: Affective Instability, Identity Problem, Negative Relationships, and Self-Harm. A score of 38 or higher suggests the presence of prominent Borderline Personality Disorder (BPD) features but not necessarily a BPD diagnosis. This measure has good internal consistency with alpha coefficients of .87, .86, and .91 for census, college, and clinical samples respectively. Test-retest reliability over 24 to 28 days was .90 and .82 for the community and college samples, respectively. Construct validity for this scale was demonstrated by correlating this measure with the MMPI, the NEO-PI and measures of object relations and substance use/abuse (Morey, 1991). The alpha coefficient for the PAI-BOR subscales in this study ranged from .66 (Identity Problems) to .83 (Affective Instability).

The Personality Diagnostic Questionnaire, 4–Borderline Personality Disorder Scale. The Personality Diagnostic Questionnaire, 4–Borderline Personality Disorder scale (PDQ-4; Hyler, 1998) consists of nine true-false items that are keyed to the eight BPD criteria listed in the Diagnostic and Statistical Manual of Mental Disorders (DSM-IV; APA, 1994). The PDQ-4 was modified such that respondents used a 4-point Likert-type scale ranging from 0 (*false, not at all true*) to 3 (*very true*). Higher scores represent greater endorsement of BPD symptoms. Adequate psychometric properties for a similar, previous version of this measure were reported (Hyler, Skodol, Oldham, & Kellman, 1992). The earlier version, the PDQ-R, has high sensitivity and moderate specificity when compared to interview measures of personality disorders (Hyler et al., 1992). The alpha coefficient for the modified PDQ-4 in this study was .79.

Procedure

Participation was anonymous. The questionnaires were randomly ordered with the exception of the Wyatt and the Demographic Information Sheet which were placed last. Participants completed the set of inventories in private rooms and then met with a researcher for debriefing. Phone numbers for university counseling services and support groups were distributed with debriefing materials.

RESULTS

Frequency of Abuse and Classification of Participants into Groups

Initially we examined the participants' responses to the Wyatt Sexual History Questionnaire. One hundred sixty-three participants (64%) reported some sort of sexual abuse prior to age 18. Fifty percent of the sample ($n = 127$) reported some sort of experience with unwanted exhibitionism; 54% percent ($n = 137$) reported unwanted touch; and 31% of the sample ($n = 79$) reported unwanted sexual interaction involving penetration.

Several methods were considered to classify participants into groups based on their Wyatt Sexual History Questionnaire responses. The first classified women who reported *any* unwanted sexual experiences before the age of 18 into the "Abuse" Group. This resulted in 64% of the sample reporting some abuse experience. Other methods of classification used penetration vs. abuse with no penetration vs. no abuse and exhibitionism only or no abuse vs. abuse. Each classification method resulted in virtually identical results, suggesting that any vs. no abuse is the most useful distinction between groups. Therefore, we will report here the results for the more liberal classification method that considered any type of unwanted sexual experience as "abuse."

We also compared the demographic characteristics of the two groups of participants. Those with a history of abuse were older (Ms = 22.07 years vs. 21.50 years) and reported more education (Ms = 14.44 years vs. 14.01 years), Fs(1,250) = 9.01 and 5.77, ps < .02, respectively. All subsequent analyses were conducted with and without age and education as covariates. The results were identical; therefore, the analyses without the covariates are presented.

Most participants were single (88.5%) and Caucasian (54.5%) or African American (33.2%); and the experience of abuse was unrelated to ethnicity or relationship status. The chi-square analysis was significant, however, for psychotherapeutic treatment (past or current), $\chi^2(N = 251, df = 1) = 8.49, p < .01$, revealing that more participants with a history of abuse (45.3%) sought treatment compared to those without a history of abuse (26.7%). It is important to note, however, that less than half of those with a history of abuse (45.3%) reported seeking treatment.

Reduction of Dependent Variables

We collected data for 25 dependent variables. We expected that many of these variables would be correlated with one another. Therefore, in an attempt to reduce the number of variables, we conducted a principal components factor analysis. A 3-factor solution accounted for 65% of the variance. We used an oblique rotation and considered variables that had a loading of .40 on a single factor to be part of that factor. Results are presented in Table 2. Two variables (YSQ-SF Overvigilance/ Inhibition and PAI-BOR Negative Relationships) did not load and one variable (PAI-BOR Identity Problems) loaded on more than one factor with this three-factor solution. These three variables were excluded from further analyses.

In order to verify that these factors were internally consistent, we created standardized (z) scores for each variable on the factor and then calculated a coefficient alpha. All alphas were acceptable (see Table 1). A mean score for each factor was calculated using the z-scores. The first

TABLE 1. Factor Loadings for Reduction of Variables and Means and Standard Deviations for the Factor Scores

		History of Abuse		No History of Abuse	
Factor 1 – Depression	α = .94	Mean	SD	Mean	SD
Variable	Factor Loading	.12	.79	−.22	.80
CDS Hopelessness	.88				
CDS Self-Criticism	.85				
CDS Helplessness	.83				
CDS Self-Blame	.74				
YSQ Autonomy/Perf	.74				
YSQ Other Directed	.72				
CDS Danger	.64				
YSQ Disconnectedness	.58				
Beck Depression Inventory	.55				
Factor 2 – Anxiety/Trauma	α = .92	Mean	SD	Mean	SD
Variable	Factor Loading	.15	.86	−.28	.68
TSC Sleep Disturbances	.89				
TSC Sexual Abuse Trauma Index	.86				
TSC Anxiety	.79				
TSC Dissociation	.75				
TSC Depression	.75				
TSC Sexual Problems	.69				
Beck Anxiety Inventory	.68				
Factor 3 – Borderline Features	· α = .88	Mean	SD	Mean	SD
Variable	Factor Loading	.13	.79	−.23	.82
PAI BOR Self-Harm	.83				
PAI BOR Impaired Limits	.72				
Personality Diagnostic Quest.	.60				
PAI BOR Affective Instability	.55				

factor was labeled "Depression," and reflects cognitive distortions, early maladaptive schemas, and symptoms of depression. The second factor was labeled "Trauma/Anxiety," and reflects trauma symptoms and generalized anxiety. The third factor was labeled "Borderline Features," and reflects symptoms of borderline personality features.

Comparison of Those with Abuse to Those Without Abuse

Three one-way general linear model (GLM) analyses were done comparing those with a history of abuse to those without such a history. Those with a history of abuse reported more depression, $F(1,252) = 10.93$, $p < .01$, $\varepsilon^2 = .04$, trauma/anxiety, $F(1,252) = 17.22$, $p < .001$, $\varepsilon^2 = .06$, and borderline personality features, $F(1,252) = 12.10$, $\varepsilon^2 = .04$ compared to those without a history of abuse (see Table 1 for means and standard deviations).

Attachment Style and History of Abuse

Initially, a one-way multivariate analysis of variance (MANOVA) was done to compare the abuse groups on the continuous variables of anxious and avoidant attachment. This revealed a significant multivariate effect, $F(2,251) = 6.58$, $p < .01$, $\varepsilon^2 = .05$. Follow-up univariate tests indicated that those with a history of abuse reported more anxious attachment ($Ms = 4.00$ vs. 3.51), $F(1, 252) = 9.12$, $p < .01$, and avoidant attachment ($Ms = 3.14$ vs. 2.71), $F(1,252) = 7.40$, $p < .01$ compared to those without a history of abuse.

A chi-square analysis was then done to examine the relationship between attachment group and whether participants reported a history of abuse. These data are presented in Table 2. This resulted in a significant $\chi^2(N = 254, df = 3) = 14.72$, $p < .01$. This analysis suggests that those with a history of abuse are more likely to have an insecure attachment style (e.g., fearful, preoccupied, and dismissing) compared to those without a history of abuse.

TABLE 2. Frequency of Attachment Style by History of Abuse

		Attachment Style				
		Secure	Fearful	Preoccupied	Dismissing	Total
No Abuse	n	41	23	24	3	91
	%	45.1	25.3	26.4	3.3	100
Abuse	n	39	55	50	19	163
	%	23.9	33.7	30.7	11.6	100

Note. Percentages are within abuse group.

Clinical Elevations and Abuse

We were interested in the degree to which a history of abuse was related to clinical elevations on several of the measures. Participants were classified into groups based on their responses to the BDI (scores ≥ 20 indicate moderate to severe depression, Beck, Steer, & Brown, 1996), BAI (scores ≥ 16 indicate moderate to severe anxiety; Beck & Steer, 1990), the CDS scales (T scores ≥ 70 indicate clinical elevations; Briere, 2000) and PAI-BOR (scores ≥ 38 indicate clinical elevations; Trull, 2001). Chi-square analyses were done to examine whether abuse history was related to clinical elevations (see Table 3). A greater proportion of CSA survivors reported clinical elevations on the BDI and BAI, χ^2 ($N = 254$, $df = 1$) = 4.12, χ^2 ($N = 254$, $df = 1$) = 13.15, respectively, $ps < .05$. Similarly, a greater proportion of CSA survivors had clinically elevated scores on the CDS Self-Blame and CDS Helplessness scales, χ^2 ($N = 254$, $df = 1$) = 4.26, χ^2 ($N = 254$, $df = 1$) = 5.26, respectively, $ps < .05$. The chi-square analyses for CDS Self-Criticism and CDS Danger revealed a trend toward a similar pattern, χ^2 ($N = 254$, $df = 1$) = 3.19, χ^2 ($N = 254$, $df = 1$) = 3.54, $ps = .07$ and .06, respectively. Finally, there was no relationship between abuse history and the PAI-BOR and CDS Hopelessness, χ^2 ($N = 254$, $df = 1$) = 2.28, χ^2 ($N = 254$, $df = 1$) = .31, respectively, $ps > .10$.

TABLE 3. Frequency of Clinical Elevations by History of Abuse

	No History of Abuse	History of Abuse
BDI	13 (14.3%)	41 (25.2%)
BAI	13 (14.3%)	58 (35.6%)
PAI-BOR	19 (20.9%)	48 (29.4%)
CDS Self Criticism	17 (18.7%)	47 (28.8%)
CDS Self Blame	21 (23.1%)	58 (35.6%)
CDS Hopeless	14 (15.4%)	21 (12.9%)
CDS Danger	18 (19.8%)	50 (30.7%)
CDS Helpless	15 (16.5%)	48 (29.4%)

Note. Percentages are within abuse group.

DISCUSSION

A significant finding in our research was the prevalence of those who reported some incidence of sexual abuse before the age of 18 (e.g., 64%). Of those who reported abuse, 33% experienced unwanted touch and exhibitionism and 31% experienced penetration. Even after removing those participants who endorsed only exhibitionism, the abuse group was still over 50%. As expected, women with a history of CSA reported more symptoms of depression, trauma/anxiety, and borderline personality features. As predicted, CSA survivors also reported more avoidant and anxious attachment. Also consistent with our hypotheses, CSA survivors were more likely to be classified as insecurely attached.

A greater proportion of CSA survivors had clinical elevations on measures of depression, anxiety, and the cognitive distortions of self-blame and helplessness. There was a trend toward a greater proportion of CSA survivors having clinical elevations on the cognitive distortions of self-criticism and danger. There was no relationship between abuse history and elevations on borderline features and the distortion of hopelessness.

Taken together, these findings indicate that CSA survivors experience more affective disturbance and more cognitive distortions compared to their non-CSA counterparts. Not surprisingly, CSA survivors experience significant self-blame and helplessness. They report more anxiety, depression, and symptoms of trauma. Survivors of CSA also report more insecure attachment in their relationships with others. They experience more discomfort with closeness as well as anxiety about their relationships. Whereas 45% of those without a history of CSA reported secure attachment, less than 24% of the CSA survivors reported secure attachment. CSA survivors were more likely to be fearful, preoccupied, and dismissing in their attachment style compared to the non-CSA survivors. Yet in spite of these emotional and interpersonal difficulties, less than half of the participants who report a history of CSA received treatment.

Although some of our effect sizes are small by conventional standards, as Ondersman et al. (2001) point out, these small effect sizes may reflect important effects for many individuals. Consistent with this perspective, approximately 10% to 20% more participants with a history of CSA displayed clinical elevations on measures of psychopathology. Therefore, despite the small statistical effect size, these findings have important clinical implications.

These findings speak to the need for heightened awareness and early intervention for CSA survivors. At the present time, prevention programs related to CSA appear to be targeted at two general populations: school-age children (e.g., Davis & Gidycz, 2000; Plummer, 2001) and those at risk of sexual offending (e.g., Blanchard & Tabachnick, 2002). Other populations less frequently targeted include parent, teachers, and the public (Plummer, 2001). It appears that prevention programs are leaving out a critical population–those who have already been abused during childhood. Our data suggest that this group of women (and we can speculate men as well) is at greater risk for affective disturbance, interpersonal problems, and psychiatric disorders. Though some would argue that secondary and tertiary prevention efforts are targeted at this population, our results indicate that only 45% of the CSA survivors sought out treatment. Optimistically, we could hope that the remaining 55% of CSA survivors were those who were asymptomatic. Our data would suggest otherwise, however. Of those survivors who had never received treatment, approximately one-quarter, depending on the measure, had moderate to severe difficulties. There is some reason for optimism in these data, however; about three-quarters of those CSA survivors who had not received treatment did *not* have clinically elevated scores. Thus, consistent with previous research (e.g., Finkelhor, 1990; Finkelhor et al., 1990; Kendall-Tackett et al., 1993), some CSA survivors may be able to avoid significant negative outcomes even without treatment. Clearly, though, there is a need to reach CSA survivors in other ways besides traditional clinical interventions.

Our data indicate that childhood sexual abuse is related to negative outcomes later in life such as anxiety, depression, borderline personality features, and problems with adult romantic attachment. In spite of the obvious risk for CSA survivors, it appears that we are targeting the majority of prevention efforts to those who are at risk of abuse and to those who are at risk for abusing. Those who have already been abused have been left out of these efforts. Unfortunately, our research indicates that these women are at heightened risk for a multitude of problems. Since the majority of CSA survivors do not receive any form of mental health services, and the programs targeted at preventing further victimization of self or others in this population are quite limited or nonexistent, a critical population continues to go underserved. It appears that this important group of trauma survivors has somehow "fallen through the cracks" of prevention and early intervention efforts. Therefore, it is essential to develop and assess such efforts to assist this population of women survivors.

REFERENCES

Alexander, P. C. (1993). The differential effects of abuse characteristics and attachment in the prediction of long-term effects of sexual abuse. *Journal of Interpersonal Violence, 8*, 346-362.

American Psychological Association (1994). *The Diagnostic and Statistical Manual of Mental Disorders, 4th edition (DSM-IV).* Washington, DC: Author.

Beck, A. T. (1990). *The Beck Anxiety Inventory.* San Antonio, TX: The Psychological Corporation.

Beck, A. T. (1996). *The Beck Depression Inventory-2nd edition.* San Antonio, TX: The Psychological Corporation.

Beck, A. T., Epstein, N., Brown, G., & Steer, R. A. (1988). An inventory for measuring clinical anxiety: Psychometric properties. *Journal of Consulting and Clinical Psychology, 56*, 893-897.

Beck, A. T., & Steer, R. A. (1990). *Manual for the Beck Anxiety Inventory.* San Antonio, TX: The Psychological Corporation.

Beck, A. T., Steer, R. A., & Brown, G. K. (1996). *Manual for the BDI-II.* San Antonio TX: The Psychological Corporation.

Blanchard, G., & Tabachnick, J. (2002).The prevention of sexual abuse: Psychological and public health perspectives. *Sexual Addiction and Compulsivity, 9*, 1-13.

Brennan, K. A., Clark, C. L., & Shaver, P. R. (1998). Self-report measure of adult attachment: An integrative overview. In J. A. Simpson & W. S. Rholes (Eds.), *Attachment theory and close relationships* (pp. 77-114). New York: Guilford Press.

Briere, J. N. (1996). *The Trauma Symptom Checklist.* Odessa, FL: Psychological Assessment Resources, Inc.

Briere, J. N. (2000). *Cognitive Distortion Scales: Professional Manual.* Odessa, FL: Psychological Assessment Resources, Inc.

Busby, D. M., Glenn, E., Steggell, G. L., & Adamson, D. (1993). Treatment issues for survivors of physical and sexual abuse. *Journal of Marital and Family Therapy, 19*, 377-392.

Dallam, S.J., Gleaves, D.H., Cepeda-Benito, A., Silberg, J.L., Kraemer, H.C., & Spiegel, D. (2001). The effects of child sexual abuse: Comment on Rind, Tromovitch, and Bauserman (1998). *Psychological Bulletin, 127*, 715-733.

Davis, M. K., & Gidycz, C. A. (2000). Child sexual abuse prevention programs: A meta-analysis. *Journal of Clinical Child Psychology, 29*, 257-265.

Elliott, D. M. (1994). Impaired object relations in professional women molested as children. *Psychotherapy, 31*, 79-86.

Elliott, D. M., & Briere, J. (1992). Sexual abuse trauma among professional women: Validating the Trauma Symptom Checklist-40 (TSC-40). *Child Abuse & Neglect, 16*, 391-398.

Finkelhor, D. (1990). Early and long-term effects of child sexual abuse: An update. *Professional Psychology, 21*, 325-330.

Finkelhor, D., & Dziuba-Leatherman, J. (1994). Victimization of children. *American Psychologist, 49*, 173-183.

Finkelhor, D., Hotaling, G., Lewis, I. A., & Smith, C. (1990). Sexual abuse in a national survey of adult men and women: Prevalence, characteristics, and risk factors. *Child Abuse and Neglect, 14*, 19-28.

Fleming, J., Mullen, P. E., Sibthorpe, B., Attewell, R., & Bammer, G. (1998). The relationship between childhood sexual abuse and alcohol abuse in women–a case control study. *Addiction, 93,* 1787-1798.

Friedrich, W. N., & Reams, R. A. (1987). Course of psychological symptoms in sexually abused young children. *Psychotherapy, 24,* 160-170.

Hall, L. A., Sachs, B., Rayens, M. K., & Lutenbacher, M. (1993). Childhood physical and sexual abuse: Their relationship with depressive symptoms in adulthood. *Child Abuse and Neglect, 25,* 317-323.

Hyler, S. E. (1998). *The Personality Diagnostic Questionnaire-4.* New York: New York State Psychiatric Institute.

Hyler, S. E., Skodol, A. E., Oldham, J. M., & Kellman, H. D. (1992). Validity of the Personality Diagnostic Questionnaire–Revised: A replication in an outpatient sample. *Comprehensive Psychiatry, 33,* 73-77.

Kendall-Tackett, K. A., Williams, L. M., & Finkelhor, D. (1993). Impact of sexual abuse on children: A review and synthesis of recent empirical studies. *Psychological Bulletin, 113,* 164-180.

Koopman, C., Gore-Felton, C. & Spiegel, D. (1997). Acute stress disorder symptoms among female sexual abuse survivors seeking treatment. *Journal of Child Sexual Abuse, 6,* 65-85.

Meichenbaum, D. (1995). *A clinical handbook/practical therapist manual: For assessing and treating adults with post-traumatic stress disorder (PTSD).* Ontario, CN: Institute Press.

Mitchell, K. J. (1999). Childhood sexual abuse and family functioning linked with eating and substance misuse. Mediated structural models. (Doctoral dissertation, University of Rhode Island, 1999). *Dissertation Abstracts International, 60,* 0559.

Morey, L. C. (1991). *Personality Assessment Inventory: Professional Manual.* Odessa, FL: Psychological Assessment Resources.

Oliver, J. E. (1993). Intergenerational transmission of child abuse: Rates, research and clinical implications. *American Journal of Psychiatry, 150,* 1315-1324.

Ondersma, S.J., Chaffin, M., Berliner, L., Cordon, I., Goodman, G.S., & Barnett, D. (2001). Sex with children is abuse: Comment on Rind, Tromovitch, and Bauserman (1998). *Psychological Bulletin, 127,* 707-714.

Plummer, C. A. (2001). Prevention of child sexual abuse: A survey of 87 programs. *Violence and Victims, 16,* 575-588.

Rind, B., Tromovitch, P., & Bauserman, R. (1998). A meta-analytic examination of assumed properties of child sexual abuse using college samples. *Psychological Bulletin, 124,* 22-53.

Saunders, B. E., Villeponteaux, L. A., Lipovsky, J. A., & Kilpatrick, D. G. (1992). Child sexual assault as a risk factor for mental disorder among women: A community survey. *Journal of Interpersonal Violence, 7,* 189-204.

Schmidt, N. B., Joiner, T. E., Young, J. E., & Telch, M. J. (1995). The Schema Questionnaire: Investigation of Psychometric Properties and the Hierarchical Structure of a Measure of Maladaptive Schemas. *Cognitive Therapy and Research, 19,* 295-321.

Sorensen, S. B., Siegel, J. M., Golding, J. M., & Stein, J. A. (1991). Repeated sexual victimization. *Victims and Violence, 91,* 299-308.

Stein, J. A., Golding, J. M., Siegel, J. M., Burnam, M. A., & Sorensen, S. B. (1988). Long-term psychological sequelae of child sexual abuse: The Los Angeles Epidemiological Catchment Area Study. In G. E. Wyatt & G. J. Powell (Eds.), *The lasting effects of child sexual abuse* (pp. 135-154). Newbury Park, CA: Sage.

Trull, T. J. (2001). Structural relations between borderline personality disorder features and putative etiological correlates. *Journal of Abnormal Psychology, 110*, 471-481.

Waller, G., Meyer, C., & Ohanian, V. (2001). Psychometric properties of the long and short versions of the Young Schema Questionnaire: Core beliefs among bulimic and comparison women. *Cognitive Therapy and Research, 25*, 137-147.

Wyatt, G. E. (1985). The sexual abuse of Afro-American and White-American women in childhood. *Child Abuse and Neglect, 9*, 507-519.

Young, J., & Brown, G. (1994). *The Young Schema Questionnaire, Short Form.* New York: Cognitive Therapy Center of New York.

Physical and Sexual Trauma, Psychiatric Symptoms, and Sense of Community Among Women in Recovery: Toward a New Model of Shelter Aftercare

Bradley D. Olson
Carmen E. Curtis
Leonard A. Jason
Joseph R. Ferrari
Elizabeth V. Horin
Margaret I. Davis
Andrea M. Flynn
Josefina Alvarez

Center for Community Research
DePaul University

SUMMARY. Innovations are needed that extend the time of care for women and children in domestic violence shelters. This study looks at

Address correspondence to: Brad Olson, Center for Community Research, DePaul University, 990 W. Fullerton, Chicago, IL 60614 (E-mail: bolson@depaul.edu).

The authors appreciate the financial support provided by NIAAA, grant AA12218-02 and NIDA, grant #DA13231. The authors also thank Lucia d'Arlach, Samuel Layne, Maria Reyes, Kimberly Roberts, and Kathy Erickson.

67

one potential model called Oxford House, a mutual-help residence that has been traditionally used for individuals recovering from substance abuse problems. This recovery home can be implemented at low cost, has no time-limited stay policies, and can provide economic independence for women and their children. To determine whether patterns of past trauma and psychiatric symptoms were comparable to those found in prior research and to examine whether female residents found Oxford House to be a therapeutic environment, adult trauma, psychiatric symptoms, and sense of community were examined. Findings indicated that adult physical trauma but not adult sexual trauma predicted lifetime depression, suicide attempts, and anxiety. These results were interpreted in relation to the learned helplessness hypothesis of why some individuals remain in abusive relationships. Participants in the study also reported high sense of community scores, and no significant differences on this measure were found between women who did and did not have a history of trauma. The potential for Oxford House as a form of aftercare to extend the length and quality of treatment for women leaving domestic violence shelters is discussed. *[Article copies available for a fee from The Haworth Document Delivery Service: 1-800-HAWORTH. E-mail address: <docdelivery@haworthpress.com> Website: <http://www.HaworthPress.com> © 2003 by The Haworth Press, Inc. All rights reserved.]*

KEYWORDS. Trauma, recovery, aftercare

Using a large representative sample, the National Institute of Justice and Center for Disease Control (NIJ/CDC) estimated that 1.5 million women are victimized by intimate partner physical abuse or intimate partner rape annually in the United States (NIJ/CDC, 2000). Even more alarming are prevalence rates suggesting that 22% of women have been physically assaulted by their partners at some point in their lives and that almost 8% have experienced intimate partner rape (NIJ/CDC). More often than not, these events occur multiple times with the same partner. Furthermore, even after leaving an abusive relationship for a safer setting, as many as 78% of women have been found to return to abusive relationships (see Strube, 1988).

Effective interventions will need to counter the forces that prevent many women from leaving abusive relationships, including economic dependence, unemployment, homelessness, fewer years of education, and the lack of other resources necessary to remain independent of an abusive partner (see Gelles, 1976; Pfouts, 1978; Sullivan, Tan, Basta, Rumptz et al., 1992; Toro et al., 1995; Strube & Barbour, 1983). Another potential barrier is substance abuse that creates a dependence not only on the drug but on other people and specific contexts in which the drug was used (see Easton, Swan, & Sinha, 1999; Stewart & Israelis, 2002; Tolman & Rosen, 2001; Werkerle & Wall, 2002). Other barriers are age and having been exposed to violence as a child (Gelles).

One of the most significant barriers an intervention would need to address is depression. Depression, for instance, is closely associated with learned helplessness, which has been offered as a theory of why many individuals remain in abusive relationships. The theory of learned helplessness suggests that a continuing lack of contingency between response and outcomes, regardless of a person's attempts to improve a relationship, leads to depression and inaction (Strube, 1988). Cognitively, individuals in this situation can acquire a negative self-perception, a lack of perceived control, and a reduced ability to cope actively in a self-protective manner (Koss, 1997). The depression/learned helplessness model is supported by several studies that have found strong relationships between trauma, depression, anxiety, and suicide attempts (Haj-Yahia, 2000; Osgood & Manetta, 2000; Zlotnick, Kohn, Peterson, & Pearlstein, 1998), and findings that feelings of powerlessness following intimate partner abuse are predictive of depression at a 6-month follow-up (Campbell, Sullivan, & Davidson, 1995).

An intervention may best counter the negative cognitive effects associated with depression and learned helplessness through the empowering effects of peer support (see Hartman, 1987; Hobfall, 1985) and life in a setting where individuals have a high sense of community that increases the cost-benefit ratio of leaving a relationship (see Bishop, Chertok, & Jason, 1997; Ferrari, Jason, Olson, Davis, & Alvarez, 2002). Indeed, studies have shown that the provision of social support, safety, and a greater accessibility to resources can increase the quality of life experienced by women in these situations (Sullivan, Tan, Basta, Rumptz et al., 1992), and have led to reductions in depression at a six-month follow-up (Tan, Basta, Sullivan, & Davidson, 1995) and a one-year follow-up (Mertin & Mohr, 2001).

A diverse array of shelter-based programs exist for women and their children who have experienced domestic violence. The majority of these shelters offer a variety of services and take rigorous security measures such as having strong entrance locks and intercom systems, and having undisclosed locations, requiring that residents take oaths to prevent them from revealing the location of the facility (Sullivan &

Gillium, 2001). These settings have the potential to provide peer support and a sense of community. Unfortunately, due to high costs to maintain the facilities and pay staff, shelters often become overcrowded, causing women to be turned away. For those who become shelter residents, policies limiting the length of stay often do not provide individuals with enough time to fully develop supportive relationships. A greater length of stay is not only likely to increase a sense of community, but may also help women better recover from other problems (e.g., substance use and depression). Nevertheless, while studies have found that many women enter a shelter with little more than the intention of obtaining a short respite from a violent relationship (Strube, 1988), the majority report having nowhere to go after leaving a shelter (Strube & Barbour, 1984). All of these factors can contribute to the high rates of returning to an assailant after discharge from a shelter (Strube). Therefore, low-cost aftercare is needed that has no time-limited stay policy, provides women with resources and economic independence, provides a sense of community, and addresses issues of substance abuse, trauma, and depression.

One such option is Oxford House (see Jason et al., 1997), a mutual-help residence that began as a home for substance abuse recovery and grew to over 850 houses in the United States, including homes for women and women with children (Olson et al., 2002). Oxford Houses are completely self-run by residents. Because residents work and pay their own rent, Oxford Houses are run at a lower cost than other independent or government-run programs, and for this reason Oxford House has no time-limited stay policy. Furthermore, this model offers residents economic independence and a sense of self-liberation. The primary reason residents report moving into Oxford House, however, is peer support (Majer, Jason, Ferrari, & North, 2001). Mutual-help settings have also been thought to be ideal for women in domestic violence situations because they are particularly effective at increasing hope, helping women take responsibility for themselves, changing their locus of control, making their coping techniques more proactive, and setting up interdependent relationships as opposed to dependent relationships with others (Hartman, 1987). In many ways, the empowerment offered by these groups is in opposition to learned helplessness. Nevertheless, we know of no residential mutual-help options set up explicitly on a shelter-based model.

Therefore, the purpose of this study is three-fold: to get a sense of the prevalence data on adult trauma of women in living in women and children's Oxford Houses, to examine whether their past history suggests patterns similar to other samples who have experienced adult trauma and psychiatric symptoms such as depression, and to assess whether women in these houses have a high sense of community. It was hypothesized that rates of trauma in this study would be comparable to other substance using populations (Easton et al., 1999). It was also predicted that, based on the learned helplessness hypothesis, and studies of trauma and psychiatric symptoms, that different forms of adult trauma (e.g., adult physical and sexual trauma) would be associated with greater psychiatric symptoms (e.g., depression). In addition, despite expected past trauma, it was predicted that women in women and children's Oxford Houses would report a high sense of community, which would suggest a positive and potentially therapeutic setting.

METHOD

Participants and Procedure

Fifty-eight participants were recruited from women and children's Oxford Houses by phone and through the mail by two clinical-community PhD graduate students. The interviewers telephoned House Presidents, informed them of the nature of the study, and sent consent forms to all houses where members expressed interest. When the interviewers received signed consent forms, they phoned the participants, and set up mutually convenient times for interviews. Participants were assured of all confidentiality guidelines, encouraged to ask questions about the study, and paid $15 after completion of the interview.

Measures

Participants were administered four reliable and valid self-report measures. The Addiction Severity Index (ASI) (see McLellan et al., 1985) was used to assess age, years of education, years of alcohol use, years of drug use (a variable calculated from reports across different specific drug categories), and history of psychiatric symptoms (i.e., depression, suicidal attempts, anxiety, and hallucinations). The Trauma History Questionnaire (Golding, 1994; see also Taylor and Jason, 2002) was used to assess lifetime occurrence of child abuse (combined sexual and physical), adult physical abuse, and adult sexual abuse. The Perceived Sense of Community Scale (PSCS), developed by Bishop et al., 1997, was also administered. The PSCS is measured on a five-point scale (higher score indicating a higher sense of community) and has three subscales: mission, reciprocal responsibility, and harmony. Finally, all participants were administered Reynolds' (1985) 13-item version of the Marlowe-Crowne Scale to examine any potential patterns of socially desirable responding.

RESULTS

Demographics and Prevalence

Roughly 850 Oxford Houses in the United States presently exist, but at the time of this study, only 15 were officially designated as women and children's houses, making roughly 125 women eligible to participate. Forty-eight percent of these potential participants were successfully recruited for the study. Participants in the sample were found to have an average age of 36 years and 12 years of education. Fifty percent of the participants were African American, 44.8% were European American, 3.4% were Latina, and one participant was Native American.

Descriptive analyses revealed that participants had substantial substance abuse histories, ranging from 37.5% who had used heroin (for an average of 9.5 years) to 92.9% who had used alcohol (for an average of 16.3 years). Cocaine use occurred in 89.1% of the sample (for an average of 11.9 years). Data on psychiatric symptoms indicated that 66.7% of the sample had experienced depression in their lifetimes, 45.6% had attempted suicide, 64.9% had experienced anxiety, and 22.8% had experienced hallucinations. The trauma results showed that 56.9% of the sample had experienced some form of childhood trauma (physical and/or sexual). Results for adult abuse indicated that 36.2% had experienced adult physical trauma and 35.1% had experienced adult sexual trauma, rates that are comparable to other samples recovering from substance abuse problems (see Easton et al., 1999).

Trauma and Psychiatric Symptoms: Logistic Regression Analysis

Four logistic regression models were used to separately predict the occurrence of lifetime depression, suicide attempts, anxiety, and hallucinations. Predictor variables in all four models included past adult physical and sexual trauma, and a set of control variables including age, years of education, years of alcohol use, years of drug use, and history of childhood trauma. The control variables were entered in the first block of the model prior to the adult trauma predictors to (a) meet the specificity assumption of logistic regression, (b) explore potential effects of these variables, and (c) control for the first block variables by also having them entered in the second block model along with adult physical trauma and adult sexual trauma.

Table 1 presents results from the logistic regression on depression. Of the variables in the first block, child history of trauma was marginally significant with $p = .06$. However, in the second block, when physical and sexual trauma and all other factors were entered in the model, the only significant logistic regression coefficient was the occurrence of adult physical trauma (see Table 1). The coefficient for adult sexual trauma, however, was not significant. Similar patterns for adult physical abuse were found with the second regression model predicting the existence of past suicide attempts (see Table 1).

Table 2 presents results from the logistic regression analysis on anxiety, which were similar to the effects found for both depression and past suicide attempts. The logistic regression analysis predicting hallucinations is also presented in Table 2, indicating that the coefficients for years of education and adult physical abuse showed marginal, albeit

TABLE 1. Logistic Regression Effects of Adult Physical Abuse and Adult Sexual Abuse on Lifetime Occurrence of Mental Disorders

| | Lifetime Occurrence | | | | | | | |
| | Depression | | | | Suicidal Attempts | | | |
Step and Predictor	β (S.E.)	Wald	p	OR	β (S.E.)	Wald	p	OR
Block 1								
Age	.03 (.04)	.61	.44	1.03	−.03 (.04)	.46	.50	.97
Years Education	−.04 (.14)	.10	.75	.96	−.01 (.12)	.00	.95	.99
Years Alcohol Use	.04 (.05)	.80	.37	1.04	.05 (.04)	1.51	.22	1.05
Years Drug Use	−.04 (.06)	.45	.50	.96	.02 (.05)	.10	.75	1.02
Child Trauma	1.23 (.66)	3.5	.06	3.4	1.48 (.66)	5.02	.03*	4.40
Block 2								
Adult Physical Trauma	2.01 (1.04)	3.74	.05*	7.46	1.84 (.90)	4.22	.04*	6.32
Adult Sexual Trauma	.69 (.80)	.74	.39	1.99	.53 (.81)	.42	.52	1.70

Note. *Highlights significant effects, $p < .05$. The significant child trauma coefficients become non-significant when the second block predictors are included in the overall model. This is largely due to the effect of adult physical abuse, suggesting it may play a mediational role in the relationship between child trauma and lifetime psychiatric symptoms.

TABLE 2. Logistic Regression Effects of Adult Physical Abuse and Adult Sexual Abuse on Lifetime Occurrence of Mental Disorders

	Lifetime Occurrence							
	Anxiety				Hallucinations			
Step and Predictor	β (S.E.)	Wald	p	OR	β (S.E.)	Wald	p	OR
Block 1								
Age	.00 (.04)	.01	.92	1.00	−.06 (.06)	1.15	.28	.94
Years Education	−.10 (.15)	.50	.48	.90	−.33 (.17)	3.56	.06	.72
Years Alcohol Use	.02 (.04)	.21	.65	1.02	.05 (.05)	.03	.31	1.06
Years Drug Use	−.02 (.05)	.13	.71	.98	−.02 (.06)	.07	.80	.98
Child Trauma	.81 (.62)	1.69	.19	2.25	.05 (.80)	.00	.95	1.05
Block 2								
Adult Physical Trauma	2.53 (1.06)	5.73	.02*	12.57	1.99 (1.10)	3.25	.07	7.29
Adult Sexual Trauma	.72 (.81)	.79	.37	2.05	−.875 (.88)	.99	.32	.42

*Highlights significant effects, $p < .05$.

non-significant, effects. As in the prior three models, sexual abuse was not a significant predictor of lifetime psychiatric symptoms.

Sense of Community: MANCOVA Analysis

Based on the hypothesis that sense of community would be high in this sample, the average mean composite and means for the three subscales were examined. These means ($M = 3.96$ for the average Perceived Sense of Community score, 4.04 for Mission, 4.07 for Reciprocal Responsibility, and 3.56 for Harmony) indicated scores that are higher than any other sample that has been reported using this instrument. For instance, across four different samples ranging from student groups, work groups, scout groups and church groups, Halamová (2001) reports an average PSCS score of 3.56. The Oxford House residents in the present sample, however, were only slightly higher than the church sample reported by Halamová, which had an average PSCS score of 3.93 (see also Bishop, Jason, Ferrari, & Huang, 1998 for yet another sample in substance abuse recovery).

We next compared those who had experienced either past adult physical or adult sexual trauma to those who had not experienced either form of trauma, and controlled for any potential social desirability biases. A

MANCOVA was employed using a 2 (no adult physical abuse, adult physical abuse) × 2 (no adult sexual abuse, adult sexual abuse) design (covarying social desirability), with the three correlated subscales of reciprocal responsibility, mission, and harmony as dependent variables. Neither the adult physical abuse main effect, Wilks' λ (3, 47) = 1.14, p = .342, the adult sexual abuse main effect Wilks' λ (3, 47) = .46, p = .71, nor the interaction, Wilks' λ (3, 47) = .77, p = .51, was significant. For exploratory purposes, correlations between psychiatric symptoms and sense of community were also obtained, although no significant relationships were found.

DISCUSSION

The findings of the present study indicate that the respondents showed substantial alcohol, drug, and trauma histories resembling rates found in studies with similar samples (Easton et al., 1999). An adult history of physical abuse predicted the past occurrence of depression, suicide attempts, and anxiety. Furthermore, while the women reported severe traumatic and emotional histories, extremely high sense of community scores were found in the sample and there were no differences in the reported level of sense of community between those who had or had not experienced trauma. These findings suggest that the Oxford House model has been able to successfully create a substantial sense of community in these residents, and that Oxford House may have the potential to afford therapeutic and empowering effects on individuals who have experienced trauma, a low sense of self-worth and dependence rather than interdependence in past relationships.

Adult physical trauma was found to predict depression and other psychiatric symptoms as has been found in other studies (Haj-Yahia, 2000; Osgood & Manetta, 2000; Zlotnick et al., 1998). The fact that adult physical abuse was a consistently stronger predictor than adult sexual abuse was an unexpected finding, particularly due to the emotional severity of sexual abuse. The differential effects for physical and sexual abuse were of additional interest because little is known about the psychological impact of varied forms of trauma (NIJ/CDC, 2002). One potential explanation for these differential effects may be found in the application of learned helplessness to trauma and relationship violence. Research suggests, for instance, that adult physical abuse tends to occur repeatedly, at a greater rate, and over a longer period of time than adult sexual abuse (NIJ/CDC, 2000) and these conditions may be necessary for learned helplessness to develop. It is possible that, due to the severity of adult sexual trauma, individuals who have been victimized in this way are more likely to permanently leave the relationship before it occurs again than those who are victimized by assaults of a purely physical nature. Thus, despite the varied harms that sexual abuse is likely to produce, the time period over which it may have occurred could have reduced the likelihood that it would be statistically associated with the depressive symptoms and cognitive effects associated with learned helplessness, particularly in this moderately small sample. In contrast, because people victimized by intimate partner physical assault are likely to remain in the relationship longer (NIJ/CDC, 2000), they have a longer time span in which to develop feelings of frustration, disillusionment, worthlessness, and related symptoms.

In addition, in contrast to physical trauma, sexual trauma is not only less likely to be repeated (on average 1.6 times [NIJ/CDC, 2000]), but is also more likely to occur in qualitatively different contexts and with different assailants (a possibility which unfortunately cannot be assessed in this study) that may have reduced its statistical association with depressive symptoms. For instance, sexual assault may occur more often in the context of purchasing narcotics where the relationship may not be as likely to continue over several years or involve as much attachment to the perpetrator.

A more methodological explanation for the lack of an effect with sexual abuse is that the definition of sexual abuse is not as likely to be the same for all people as is the case with physical abuse, leading participants to underreport the occurrence of sexual trauma and thereby obscuring its relationship with psychiatric symptoms. For instance, an event that is by every other definition traumatic would be less likely to be reported by the participant as sexual abuse if it occurred in the exchange of sex for drugs or if it occurred within the context of a marriage. Certainly, more research needs to be conducted on the effects of different forms of trauma on psychiatric symptoms.

The present study also found high sense of community scores for women with and without past trauma. This finding suggests that, despite past difficulties, Oxford House has provided a positive, community-based setting for these women–one that is likely to impart active coping skills and provide the supportive relationships that can diminish feelings of helplessness and other emotions associated with depression.

Clearly, domestic violence shelters play an important role in the health care system, but gaps exist in services provided to those victimized by intimate partner violence and other forms of abuse. Researchers have suggested that these services could be improved through the provision of low-cost aftercare that offers social support, employment, housing (Sullivan, Basta, Tan, & Davidson, 1992), security, physical protection (Mertin & Mohr, 2001), the modeling of more effective coping strategies (Brown & O'Brien, 1998), a responsive environment for children (Sullivan & Gillium, 2001), and a greater integration of services with substance abuse treatment (Collins, Kroutil, Roland, & Moore-Guerrara, 1997; Bennet & Lawson, 1994; Werkerle & Wall, 2002).

For individuals who leave shelters with few housing opportunities, a modified Oxford House model may be an attractive option. Unlike domestic violence shelters, many Oxford Houses have a seeming disadvantage of being located in the center of residential neighborhoods without intercoms and other security measures at their entrances. When a person is voted into an Oxford House, however, residents obtain information about the new resident's past troublesome relationships (e.g., the name of a past perpetrator), and this information is used to protect all residents, particularly those who have been threatened or are known to be in immediate danger.

In addition to security, domestic violence shelters offer a greater array of programs than Oxford House including counseling for trauma, depression and related issues, all of which are likely to help women successfully work toward remaining independent of an abusive setting. Oxford House, however, also encourages residents to seek professional help outside the home, and the mutual-help nature of the setting provides informational and emotional support that holds many of the therapeutic benefits offered in professional therapies for depression and other psychiatric symptoms such as post-traumatic stress disorder (Olson et al., 2002). Therefore, once women have spent time in a domestic violence shelter and are ready for greater independence, they would benefit from an option such as Oxford House where they can extend their length of care in a more self-governing setting. Oxford House as shelter aftercare may be one of the most effective models to alleviate the economic burden on shelters, thereby freeing up the shelters' resources so that the facility may serve an increasing number of women and children in need of immediate services.

REFERENCES

Bennet, L., & Lawson, M. (1994). Barriers to cooperation between domestic violence and substance-abuse programs. *Family in Society*, *75*, 277-286.

Bishop, P. D., Chertok, F., & Jason, L. A. (1997). Measuring a sense of community: Beyond local boundaries. *Journal of Primary Prevention*, *18*, 193-212.

Bishop, P. D., Jason, L. A., Ferrari, J. R., & Huang, C. F. (1998). A survival analysis of communal-living self-help, addiction recovery participants. *American Journal of Community Psychology*, *26*, 803-821.

Brown, C. & O'Brien, K. M. (1998). Understanding stress and burnout in shelter workers. *Professional Psychology: Research & Practice*, *29(4)*, 383-385.

Campbell, R., Sullivan, C. M., & Davidson, W. S. (1995). Women who use domestic violence shelters: Changes in depression over time. *Psychology of Women Quarterly*, *19(2)*, 237-255.

Collins, J., Kroutil, L., Roland, J., & Moore-Gurrera, M. (1997). Issues on the linkages of alcohol and domestic violence services. In M. Galanter (Series Ed.), *Recent developments in alcoholism, Vol. 13: Alcohol and violence: Epidemiology, neurobiology, psychology, family issues* (pp. 387-405). Plenum Press.

Easton, C., Swan, S., & Sinha, R. (1999). Prevalence of family violence in clients entering substance abuse treatment. *Journal of Substance Abuse*, *12*, 641-654.

Ferrari, J. R., Jason, L. A., Olson, B. D., Davis, M., & Alvarez, J. (2002). Sense of community among Oxford House residents recovering from substance abuse: Making a house a home. In A. Fisher (Ed.), *Psychological Sense of Community: Research, Applications, and Implications*. New York: Kluwer-Plenum, Inc.

Gelles, R. J. (1976). Abused wives: Why do they stay? *Journal of Marriage and the Family*, *38*, 659-668.

Golding, J. M. (1994). Sexual assault history and physical health in randomly selected Los Angeles women. *Health Psychology*, *13*, 130-138.

Haj-Yahia, M. (2000). Implications of wife abuse and battering for self-esteem, depression, and anxiety. *Journal of Family Issues*, *21*, 435-463.

Halamová, J. (2001). Psychological Sense of Community: Examining McMillian-Chavis' and Peck's concepts. *Studia Psychologica*, *43*, 137-148.

Hartman, S. (1987). Therapeutic self-help group: A process of empowerment for women in abusive relationships. In C. M. Brody (Ed.), *Women's therapy groups: Paradigms of feminist treatment* (pp. 67-81). New York: Springer.

Hobfall, S. E. (1985). *Stress, Social Support, & Women*. New York: McGraw-Hill.

Jason, L. A., Ferrari, J. R., Smith, B., Marsh, P., Dvorchak, P. A., & Groessl, E. J. et al. (1997). An exploratory study of male recovering substance abusers living in a self-help, self-governed setting. *The Journal of Mental Health Administration*, *24*, 332-339.

Koss, M. P. (1997). The Women's mental health research agenda: Violence against women. The Lanahan Readings in the Psychology of Women (Ed., Toni-Ann Roberts). Baltimore: Lanahan Publishers, Inc.

Majer, J. M., Jason, L. A., Ferrari, J. R., & North, C. S. (2001). Comorbidity among Oxford House residents: A preliminary outcome study. *Addictive Behaviors*, *26*, 1-9.

McLellan, A. T., Luborsky, L., Cacciola, J., Griffith, J., Evans, F., Barr, H., & O'Brien, C. P. (1985). New data from the Addiction Severity Index: Reliability and validity in three centers. *Journal of Nervous and Mental Disease, 173,* 412-423.

Mertin, P. & Mohr, P. B. (2001). A follow-up study of posttraumatic stress disorder, anxiety, and depression in Australian victims of domestic violence. *Violence & Victims, 16(6),* 645-654. Springer Publishing, US, www.springerpub.com.

National Institute of Justice/Center for Disease Control. (2000). Extent, nature, and consequences of intimate partner violence: Findings from the national violence against women survey.

O'Farrell, T., & Feehan, M. (1999). Alcoholism treatment and the family: Do the family and individual treatments for alcoholic adults have preventive effects for children? *Journal of Studies on Alcohol, 13,* 125-129.

Olson, B. D., Jason, L. A., d'Arlach, L., Ferrari, J. R., Alvarez, J., Davis, M. I., Olabode-Dada, O., Horin, E., Oleniczak, J., Cooper, D. G., Burger, T. N., Curtis, C., Flynn, A. M., Sasser, K. C., & Viola, J. J. (2002). Oxford House, Second-Order Thinking, and the Diffusion of Systems-Based Innovations. *The Community Psychologist, 35(2),* 20-22.

Olson, B. D., Jason, L. A., Ferrari, J. R., & Hutcheson, T. D. (2002). *Bridging Professional- and Mutual-Help Through a Unifying Theory of Change: An Application of the Transtheoretical Model to the Mutual-Help Organization.* Manuscript submitted for publication.

Osgood, N. J., & Manetta, A. A. (2000). Abuse and suicidal issues in older women. *Journal of Death and Dying, 42,* 71-81.

Pfouts, J. H. (1978). Violent families: Coping responses of abused wives. *Child Welfare, 57,* 101-111.

Reynolds, W. M. (1982). Development of reliable and valid short forms of the Marlowe-Crowne Social Desirability Scale. *Journal of Clinical Psychology, 38,* 119-125.

Stewart, S., & Isreali, A. L. (2002). Substance abuse and co-occurring psychiatric disorders in victims of inmate violence. In C. Werkerle (Ed.), *The violence and addiction equation* (pp. 98-122). New York: Brunner-Routledge.

Strube, M. J. (1988). The decision to leave an abusive relationship: Empirical evidence and theoretical issues. *Psychological Bulletin, 104,* 236-250.

Strube, M. J. & Barbour, L. S. (1983). The decision to leave an abusive relationship: Economic dependence and psychological commitment. *Journal of Marriage and the Family, 46,* 785-793.

Sullivan, C. M., Tan, C., Basta, J. & Rumptz, M. et al. (1992). An advocacy intervention program for women with abusive partners: Initial evaluation. *American Journal of Community Psychology, 20(3),* 309-332.

Sullivan, C. M. & Gillium, T. (2001). Shelters and other community-based services for battered women and their children. In C. M. Renzetti & J. L. Edleson (Eds.), *Sourcebook on violence against women* (pp. 247-260). Thousand Oaks, CA: Sage Publications.

Sullivan, C. M., Basta, J., Tan, C., & Davidson, W. S. (1992). After the crisis: A needs assessment of women leaving a domestic violence shelter. *Violence & Victims, 7(3),* 267-275.

Taylor, R. R. & Jason, L. A. (2002). Sexual abuse, physical abuse, chronic fatigue, and Chronic Fatigue Syndrome: A community-based study. *Journal of Nervous and Mental Disease.*

Tolman, R. M, & Rosen, D. (2001). Domestic violence in the lives of women receiving welfare. *Violence Against Women, 7(2)*, 141-158.

Toro, P., Bellavia, C., & Daeschler, C. et al. (1995). Distinguishing homelessness from poverty: A comparative study. *Journal of Consulting & Clinical Psychology, 63*, 280-289.

Wekerle, C. & Wall, A. (2002). *The violence and addiction equation: Theoretical and clinical issues in substance abuse and relationship violence.* New York: Brunner-Routledge.

Zlotnick, C., Kohn, R., Peterson, D., & Pearlstein, T. (1998). Partner physical victimization in a national sample of American families: Relationship to psychological functioning, psychosocial factors, and gender. *Journal of Interpersonal Violence, 13(1)*, 156-166.

The Relationship Between Attachment Styles and Vicarious Traumatization in Female Trauma Therapists

Elizabeth Marmaras
Sandra S. Lee

Seton Hall University
South Orange, NJ

Harold Siegel

Rutgers the State University
Newark, NJ

Warren Reich

Iona College
New Rochelle, NY

SUMMARY. This study explores the role of attachment styles in vicarious traumatization in a national sample of 375 female therapists who

Address correspondence to: Elizabeth Marmaras, PhD (E-mail: Emarmaras@aol.com).
The data reported here were part of the data collected for Elizabeth Marmaras' doctoral dissertation, which was supervised by Sandra Lee, PhD, in the Department of Professional Psychology and Family Therapy, Seton Hall University, South Orange, NJ 07079.

[Haworth co-indexing entry note]: "The Relationship Between Attachment Styles and Vicarious Traumatization in Female Trauma Therapists." Marmaras, Elizabeth et al. Co-published simultaneously in *Journal of Prevention & Intervention in the Community* (The Haworth Press, Inc.) Vol. 26, No. 1, 2003, pp. 81-92; and: *Traumatic Stress and Its Aftermath: Cultural, Community, and Professional Contexts* (ed: Sandra S. Lee) The Haworth Press, Inc., 2003, pp. 81-92. Single or multiple copies of this article are available for a fee from The Haworth Document Delivery Service [1-800-HAWORTH, 9:00 a.m. - 5:00 p.m. (EST). E-mail address: docdelivery@haworthpress.com].

10.1300/J005v26n01_07

work with adult outpatient trauma survivors. Participants completed measures of attachment styles and vicarious traumatization. Multiple regression analyses revealed a significant positive relationship between attachment styles and disrupted cognitive schemas as well as a significant positive relationship between attachment styles and symptoms of intrusion, hyperarousal and avoidance in female trauma therapists. The fearful-avoidant attachment style was the best predictor of both the cognitive disruptions and symptoms of distress in female trauma therapists. The empirical findings of this study offer important applied clinical implications for female therapists who work with adult trauma survivors. *[Article copies available for a fee from The Haworth Document Delivery Service: 1-800-HAWORTH. E-mail address: <docdelivery@haworthpress.com> Website: <http://www.HaworthPress.com> © 2003 by The Haworth Press, Inc. All rights reserved.]*

KEYWORDS. Attachment, vicarious traumatization

Survivors of traumatic events including childhood abuse, rape, domestic violence, war, and genocide have sought psychotherapy mainly in the last two decades. Since then, therapists have devoted much attention to the psychological consequences of the traumatic experiences on trauma survivors (Briere & Runtz, 1988; Figley, 1995; Herman, 1997; McCann & Pearlman, 1990; Terr, 1990).

Therapists who treat trauma survivors may experience powerful psychological effects (Herman, 1997). Furthermore, therapists who help trauma survivors open themselves to a deep personal transformation. This transformation may include personal growth, such as an increased personal awareness and a deeper connection with others, as well as psychological disruptions in the self that may be similar to post traumatic symptoms experienced by trauma survivors (McCann & Pearlman, 1990). McCann and Pearlman (1990) conceptualized the term vicarious traumatization.

The vicarious traumatization phenomenon has been labeled secondary traumatic stress disorder (STSD) (Figley, 1995) and traumatic countertransference (Herman, 1997). Vicarious traumatization, as defined by McCann and Pearlman (1990) and Pearlman and Saakvitne (1995), includes the symptomatology of secondary traumatic stress disorder as well as profound changes in the therapist's frame of reference.

Initial studies on secondary traumatic symptoms in therapists focused on therapists who worked with combat veterans and Holocaust survivors (Haley, 1974). Since then most of the empirical studies on vicarious traumatization have focused on therapists who treated survivors of sexual abuse. These studies have examined various factors including: therapists' personal history of trauma, gender, percentage of trauma survivors in caseload, number of hours spent in trauma work, number of years of professional trauma experience, therapists' involvement in their own personal therapy (Brady, Guy, Poelstra & Brokaw, 1999; Chrestman, 1995; Follette, Polusny, & Milbeck, 1994; Pearlman & MacIan, 1995; Shauben & Frazier, 1995).

The results of some studies (Brady, Guy, Poelstra & Brokaw, 1999) indicated that the therapists' symptoms of avoidance and intrusion were directly related to their current and cumulative exposure to sexual trauma survivors. These symptoms were not found in therapists working with non-trauma populations, thus further supporting the notion that vicarious traumatization is a unique phenomenon associated with treating trauma survivors (Pearlman & MacIan, 1995).

Chrestman (1995) found that increased professional experience, utilization of additional training, lower percentages of trauma cases, and higher percentages of time spent in research activities were all associated with lower distress in therapists. Higher percentages of time spent in general clinical activities was associated with increased avoidance symptoms.

ATTACHMENT AND VICARIOUS TRAUMATIZATION

Pearlman and Saakvitne (1995) proposed that therapists characteristics may interact with therapists' exposure to trauma material and may cause vicarious traumatization. These therapists' characteristics include: interpersonal style, professional development, personal trauma history and current support systems. Despite the proliferation of studies examining the role of therapists' personal trauma history, some aspects of professional development, and social support (Follette, Polusny, & Milbeck, 1994; Pearlman & Saakvitne, 1995; Shauben & Frazier, 1995), research conducted examining the relationship between therapists' interpersonal style and vicarious traumatization is sparse (Pearlman & MacIan, 1995).

According to Bowlby (1973), attachment is the foundation on which personality is built. Children internalize experiences with caretakers in such a way that attachment patterns are incorporated into the personality structure, forming internal working models of the self and others. Secure attachment enhances not only healthy interpersonal relationships, feelings of personal worth and self-efficacy, but also an individual's ability to deal with trauma. These abilities and feelings may increase the development of positive, constructive strategies for dealing with stressors, thereby resulting in improved emotional adjustment and less traumatic symptomatology (Hazan & Shaver, 1987).

Bartholomew (1991) extended work on attachment styles by positing a four-category model of attachment that empirically validates Bowlby's theory of internal working models of both self and self in relation to others. The four patterns (styles) are secure, preoccupied, fearful-avoidant, and dismissive.

Early empirical studies on attachment styles (Cashdon, 1988; Marshall & Marshall, 1988; Ricks, 1974) supported the concept that attachment organization is related to therapists' intervention intensity and to their ability to deal with vicarious trauma symptoms. Later studies (Dozier, Cue & Barnett, 1994) indicated that therapists with a secure attachment style were more attentive and responsive to the underlying needs of their insecure clients. Additionally, insecure therapists felt more distressed in their work with clients, which further implicated their ability to be responsive and attentive to them. These therapists perceived greater dependency needs and intervened more intensively. The purpose of the present study was to determine the relationship between attachment styles and vicarious traumatization.

Hypothesis one: It was hypothesized that a significant relationship would be found between the attachment styles (secure, fearful-avoidant, preoccupied and dismissive-avoidant) as measured by the Relationship Questionnaire (RQ; Bartholomew & Horowitz, 1991) and overall disrupted cognitive schemas as measured by the Traumatic Stress Institute Belief Scale (TSI; Pearlman & Saakvitne, 1994). Specifically the fearful-avoidant attachment style would be the best predictor of overall disrupted cognitive schemas.

Hypothesis two: It was hypothesized that a significant relationship would be found between the attachment styles as measured by the Relationship Questionnaire (RQ; Bartholomew & Horowitz, 1991) and symptoms of hyperarousal, intrusion and avoidance as measured by the Impact of Event Scale-Revised (IES-R; Weiss & Marmar, 1995). Specifically the fearful-avoidant attachment style will be the best predictor of hyperarousal, intrusion and avoidance symptoms.

METHOD

Subjects

A total of three hundred seventy-five female therapists who worked with adult outpatient trauma survivors participated in the study. Participants filled out a demographic questionnaire. Of the 375 female therapists, 351 (93.6%) were Caucasian, 9 (2.4%) were Hispanic, 6 (1.6%) were Native American, 4 (1.1%) were Asian, 3 (.8%) were African American, and 2 (.5%) were of other ethnic backgrounds. The most frequently represented age among the female trauma therapists was 46-55 years old (48.3%). This was followed by 36-45 years old (20.5%), 56-65 years old (20.3%), 25-35 years old (8%), and by 66 years or older (2.9%). The majority of the female trauma therapists, 72.5% held a PhD in psychology, 11.7% an MA/MS, 9.6% a PsyD, 5.1% an EdD and 1.1% held an MD. Of the female therapists, 27.7% had 11-15 years of experience working with outpatient adult trauma survivors, 24.5% had 16-20 years of trauma experience, 21.3% had 6-10 years of trauma experience, 18.1% had more than 21 years of experience and 8.3% had 1-5 years of professional experience treating adult trauma survivors. A total of 42.1% of the female trauma therapists were trauma survivors, and 57.9% were not; 78.9% were in personal therapy and 21.1% were not engaged in personal therapy at the time of this study.

Measures

The *Relationship Questionnaire* (RQ; Bartholomew & Horowitz, 1991) was used to measure the attachment style in female therapists who treat adult outpatient trauma survivors. It is a four-item self-report measure that consists of short paragraphs describing four attachment styles as they apply to close relationships in general. Each participant is asked for four scores, one for each attachment pattern, and to rate how well he or she corresponds to each prototype. The RQ was developed in the context of the four-prototype model of adult attachment (Bartholomew & Horowitz, 1991) and it allows for the measurement of the four attachment categories as well as the underlying attachment poles, view of self and view of other.

Results of the first study conducted to validate this instrument indicated high convergent validity coefficients (.34, .39, .50) and low discriminant validity coefficients (.03, −.09, −.21) (Bartholomew & Horowitz, 1991). Results of the second study also indicated both convergent validity (.41, .34, .21). and discriminant validity (.12, −.05, −.20) (Bartholomew & Horowitz, 1991).

The Trauma Stress Institute Belief Scale–Revision L (TSI Belief Scale; Pearlman & Saakvitne, 1994) was used to measure disrupted schemas in female therapists. The version of the scale used in this study is Revision L and it is an 80 item self-report that provided an overall score measuring disrupted cognitive schemas on ten subscales.

Internal consistencies (Cronbach's alphas) for the subscales (Revision L) were as follows: self-safety = .83; other-safety = .73; self-esteem = .87; other-esteem = .75; self-trust = .87; other-trust = .86; self-intimacy = .79; other-intimacy = .86; self-control = .82 and other-control = .73 (Pearlman, 1996).

The Impact of Event Scale–Revised (IES-R; Weiss & Marmar, 1995) was used to measure the behavioral symptoms of hyperarousal, intrusion and avoidance in female therapists. The IES-R is a 22-item self-report scale consisting of three subscales measuring symptoms of intrusion, avoidance and hyperarousal. It produces three scores, one for each scale, and a total score. Subjects were asked to rate the degree of distress they experienced as a result of their exposure to traumatic events within the last seven days. Responses are scored on a four-point Likert scale with anchors ranging from "0" (not at all), to "1" (rarely) to "3" (sometimes) to "5" (often).

Reliability coefficients range from .90 to .94. Internal consistency coefficients are: intrusion = .57; avoidance = .51; and hyperarousal = .59 (Weiss & Marmar, 1995). The test-retest correlation coefficients are: intrusion = .94; avoidance = .89; and hyperarousal = .92 (Weiss & Marmar, 1993). The TSI Belief Scale correlates significantly with the IES-Revised, suggesting that disrupted cognitive schemas as measured by the TSI do in fact covary with traumatic stress and dysfunction (Pearlman & MacIan, 1995).

RESULTS

The correlation coefficients between the dependent variables (disrupted cognitive schemas, symptoms of hyperarousal, intrusion and avoidance) and the independent variables (attachment styles) are presented in Table 1.

The results of a multiple regression analysis indicated a significant positive relationship between attachment styles as measured by the Relationship Questionnaire (RQ; Bartholomew & Horowitz, 1991) and

TABLE 1. Correlation Coefficients Between Dependent and Independent Variables (N = 375)

	SEC	FEAR	PREO	DIS
SEC	1.00	−.48**	−.29**	.27**
FEAR	−.48**	1.00	.23**	.16**
PREO	−.29**	.23**	1.00	.01
DIS	−.27**	.16**	.01	1.00
TSI	−.34**	.42**	.36**	.20**
IES	−.20**	.27**	.23**	.23**

	VT_TSI	VT_IES
SEC	−.34**	−.20**
FEAR	.42**	.27**
PREO	.36**	.23**
DIS	.20**	.23**
TSI	1.00	.58**
IES	.58**	1.00

Note. $*p < .05$ $**p < .01$

overall disrupted cognitive schemas in female trauma therapists as measured by the Traumatic Stress Institute Belief Scale (TSI; Pearlman & Saakvitne, 1994). Attachment styles accounted for 28% of the variance in disrupted cognitive schemas in female therapists who work with adult trauma survivors ($F = 36.66$, df = (4, 370), $p = .00$).

Visual inspection of the standardized beta coefficients (see Table 2) indicated that the fearful-avoidant and the preoccupied attachment styles showed approximately the same size relationship to disruptions in cognitive schemas ($B = .30$, $p = .00$ for the fearful-avoidant attachment style and $B = .27$ for the preoccupied attachment style). The dismissive-avoidant attachment style indicated a net relationship that is about half that size ($B = .13$, $p = .00$). The secure attachment style showed no significant relationship to disruptions in cognitive schemas on the TSI in female trauma therapists who work with outpatient trauma survivors.

The results of the second multiple regression analysis indicated that there is a significant positive relationship between attachment styles and symptoms of intrusion, avoidance and hyperarousal ($F = 15.68$, df = (4, 370), $p = .00$). Attachment styles (secure, fearful-avoidant, dismissive-avoidant, and preoccupied) accounted for 15% of the variance in symptoms of intrusion, hyperarousal and avoidance in female trauma therapists.

Visual inspection of the standardized beta coefficients (see Table 3) indicated that the fearful-avoidant was the best predictor (B = 21, p = .00) of the variability in behavioral symptoms of intrusion, avoidance and hyper arousal on the IES in female trauma therapists. However, the pre-occupied and dismissive-avoidant attachment styles showed approximately the same size relationship to symptoms of intrusion, avoidance and hyper arousal on the IES in female trauma therapists (B = .20, p = .00 for the dismissive-avoidant attachment style and B = .18, p = .00 for the preoccupied attachment style). The secure attachment style showed no significant relationship to these symptoms.

DISCUSSION

The present study utilized four attachment styles: secure, fearful-avoidant, dismissive-avoidant and preoccupied (Bartholomew & Horowitz, 1991) to

TABLE 2. Summary of the Multiple Regression Analysis of Disrupted Cognitive Schemas and Attachment Styles (N = 375)

Independent Variable	B	t	p
SEC	−.08	−1.51	.13
DIS	.13	2.94	.00
FEAR	.30	5.90	.00
PREO	.27	5.89	.00

TABLE 3. Summary of the Multiple Regression Analysis of Vicarious Traumatization Symptoms and Attachment Styles (N = 375)

Independent Variable	B	t	p
SEC	.00	.14	.88
DIS	.20	3.94	.00
FEAR	.21	3.75	.00
PREO	.18	3.62	.00

investigate whether the Fearful attachment style was the best predictor of vicarious traumatization in female therapists who work with adult trauma survivors.

Hypothesis One. The results of the study confirmed the first hypothesis and indicated a significant relationship between disrupted cognitive schemas and attachment styles. The findings indicated that female trauma therapists with a fearful or a preoccupied attachment style reported more disruptions in their cognitive schemas than female trauma therapists with a dismissive-avoidant attachment style and that trauma therapists with a secure attachment style reported very minimal cognitive disruptions.

The results of this hypothesis may be supported by the findings of Dozier, Cue and Barnett (1994) who proposed that secure case managers were able to attend and respond to their clients' needs and to use their countertransference reactions by reflecting back and intervening in ways that might have been uncomfortable to them. On the other hand, insecure case managers (those with fearful-avoidant, preoccupied or dismissive-avoidant attachment style) became very distressed in the context of the therapeutic relationship and were unable to process and use their countertransference. This inability to process their countertransference reactions subsequently might have had a negative effect on them, their clients and overall the therapeutic relationship.

The findings of this hypothesis may also be similar to findings by Shaver, Collins and Clark (1966) who reported that individuals with secure attachment styles were willing to report and to acknowledge low levels of emotional distress. In contrast, individuals with preoccupied and fearful attachment styles reported exaggerated levels of negative emotions and symptoms, whereas individuals with a dismissive style denied their feelings of distress. According to Bartholomew and Horowitz (1991), individuals with a fearful-avoidant or a preoccupied attachment style struggle with their own sense of identity, with self-regulation and with appropriate boundary setting, while individuals with a preoccupied attachment style have conflictual feelings about intimacy and closeness in interpersonal relationships.

Thus, in the current study, the female trauma therapists with a secure attachment style may have reported minimal cognitive disruptions in comparison to those with a fearful-avoidant, preoccupied, or dismissive-avoidant attachment style due to their comfort level with intimate relationships and intense emotions.

Hypothesis Two. One way to view the results of the second hypothesis is from the perspective of relational disturbances suffered by trauma therapists when they are exposed to trauma content. Herman (1997) stated that the therapists' response to the trauma survivor might be detachment, distancing and/or identification with the trauma survivor. Distancing or excessive detaching emotionally from the trauma survivor may enable the trauma worker to deal with his or her feelings of vulnerability, hopelessness, anger, fear of closeness and intimacy by blocking out such emotional reactions. Overidentification with the trauma survivor is the therapists' attempt to gain control of overwhelming feelings in the therapeutic context. Thus, the fearful-avoidant, preoccupied and dismissive-avoidant female trauma therapists in the present study who might have exhibited conflicts in interpersonal situations have reported more symptoms of hyperarousal, avoidance and intrusion.

Another way to view these results is from the perspective of individual differences in attachment styles in terms of the model of the self and model of others and its respective variations in emotional regulation and emotional expression. It appears that the female therapists in the present study with a negative view of themselves and with pre-existing difficulties in self-regulation with others (with a fearful or a preoccupied attachment style) reported more symptoms of hyperarousal, avoidance and intrusion than those female therapists with a positive view of themselves (with a secure or a dismissive-avoidant style). The results of the present study are supported by the findings of Dozier, Cue and Barnett (1994). Thus, in this study, the female trauma therapists who reported a fearful-avoidant, preoccupied or dismissive attachment style might possibly have displayed an impaired ability to evaluate the therapeutic relationship and thus be subject to more vulnerabilities, such as symptoms of hyperarousal, intrusion and avoidance. On the other hand, secure female trauma therapists may have reported minimal symptoms, as a result of their comfort with their attachment relationships to the trauma survivors and with the intense emotions activated in treatment. The sample of female trauma therapists in this study might have had a heightened degree of personal awareness, increased ability to deal with intense emotions in the therapeutic context, and the capability to take preventive measures to deal with their distress.

The findings of the present study with respect to attachment and vicarious traumatization may provide a theoretical framework to understand the effects of vicarious traumatization from a developmental perspective. The overall implications of these findings may be that therapists with unresolved issues and interpersonal difficulties may hinder the therapeutic process and be less effective in intervening.

The theoretical perspectives and empirical findings of the current study offer important applied clinical implications for female therapists who work with adult trauma survivors. One of the implications includes the importance of a multidimensional preventive approach based on physical, psychological, and interpersonal components in an effort to reduce and/or eliminate the impact of vicarious traumatization on trauma therapists. Another implication is that trauma therapists continue to assess the adequacy of their training in trauma therapy, receive supervision and/or consultation on their trauma cases, have balance and diversity in their case loads, receive social support and a confidential and professional supportive structure within which to process the impact of their work on their own personal and professional lives. Increased awareness of the impact of vicarious traumatization will also enable supervisors and other agency administrators to consider preventive approaches such as the possibility of support groups and in-service training on working with trauma survivors and on the importance of self-care of the therapists. It is also important that educational institutions incorporate in their curricula training that includes an understanding of the effects of psychological trauma, attention to countertransference and vicarious traumatization so that beginning therapists are more aware and equipped to deal with the hazards of vicarious traumatization. Lastly, an important implication is that trauma therapists consider personal therapy or some other appropriate avenue to process the feelings induced in them by trauma survivors and to discuss candidly the interface between their own experiences, their countertransference and vicarious traumatization.

Future studies need to employ the use of multiple instruments and/or interviews to measure vicarious traumatization, qualitative measures of vicarious traumatization in therapist-trauma survivor dyads, and the measurement of the impact of vicarious traumatization on treatment and/or treatment outcome and on therapists' family life and relationships.

REFERENCES

Bartholomew, K. & Horowitz, L.M. (1991). Attachment styles among young adults: A test of a four-category model. *Journal of Personality and Social Psychology, 61,* 226-244.

Bowlby, J. (1973). The making and breaking of affectional bonds. *British Journal of Psychiatry, 130,* 201-210.

Brady, P.L., Guy, J.D., Poelstra, P.L., & Brokaw, B.F. (1999). Vicarious traumatization, spirituality, and the treatment of sexual abuse survivors. A national survey of women psychotherapists. *Professional Psychology: Research and Practice, 30* (4), 386-393.

Briere, J., & Runtz, M. (1988). Symptomatology associated with childhood sexual victimization in a nonlinear adult sample. *Child Abuse and Neglect, 12,* 51-59.

Cashdon, S. (1988). Stage two: Projective identification. *Object relations therapy* (pp. 96-118). New York: Norton.

Chrestman, K.R. (1995). Secondary exposure to trauma and self reported distress among therapists. In B.H. Stamm (Ed.), *Secondary traumatic stress: Self-care issues for clinicians, researchers, and educators* (pp. 29-36). Lutherville, MD: Sidran Press.

Dozier, M., Cue, K.L., & Barnett, L. (1994). Clinicians as caregivers. Role of attachment organization in treatment. *Journal of Consulting and Clinical Psychology, 62,* 793-800.

Figley, C.R. (1995). Compassion fatigue: Toward a new understanding of the costs of caring. In B.H. Stamm (Ed.), *Secondary traumatic stress: Self-care issues for clinicians, researchers, and educators* (pp. 3-28). Lutherville, MD: Sidran Press.

Follette, V.M., Polusny, M.M. & Milbeck, K. (1994). Mental health and law enforcement professionals: Trauma history, psychological symptoms, and impact of providing services to child sexual abuse survivors. *Professional Psychology: Research and Practice, 25,* 275-282.

Haley, S.A. (1974). When the patient reports atrocities. *Archives of General Psychiatry, 30,* 191-196.

Hazan, C., & Shaver, P. (1987). Romantic love conceptualized as an attachment process. *Journal of Personality and Social Psychology, 52,* 511-524.

Herman, J.L. (1997). *Trauma and recovery.* New York: Basic Books.

McCann, I.L. & Pearlman, L.A. (1990). *Psychological trauma and the adult survivor.* New York: Brunner/Mazel.

Pearlman, L.A. & MacIan, P.S. (1995). Vicarious traumatization. An empirical study of the effects of trauma work on trauma therapists. *Professional Psychology: Research and Practice, 26,* 558-565.

Pearlman, L.A. & Saakvitne, K.W. (1995). *Trauma and the therapist: Countertransference and vicarious traumatization in psychotherapy with incest survivors.* New York: W.W. Norton & Company.

Ricks, D.F. (1974). Supershrink: Methods of a therapist judged successful on the basis of adult outcomes of adolescent patients. In D.F. Ricks, A. Thomas & M. Roff (Eds.). *Life history in psychopathology* (pp. 275-297). Minneapolis, MN: University of Minnesota Press.

Shauben, L.J. & Frazier, P.A. (1995). Vicarious trauma: The effects on female counselors on working with sexual violence survivors. *Psychology of Women Quarterly, 19,* 49-64.

Terr, L.C. (1990). What happens to early memories of trauma? *Journal of the American Academy of Child and Adolescent Psychiatry, 1,* 96-104.

Weiss, D.S. & Marmar, C.R. (1995). The Impact of Event Scale-Revised. In J.P. Wilson & Keane (Eds.), *Assessing psychological trauma and PTSD. A handbook for practitioners.* New York: Guilford Press.

Prevention in Community Mental Health Centers, edited by Robert E. Hess, PhD, and John Morgan, PhD* (Vol. 7, No. 2, 1990). *"A fascinating bird's-eye view of six significant programs of preventive care which have survived the rise and fall of preventive psychiatry in the U.S." (British Journal of Psychiatry)*

Protecting the Children: Strategies for Optimizing Emotional and Behavioral Development, edited by Raymond P. Lorion, PhD* (Vol. 7, No. 1, 1990). *"This is a masterfully conceptualized and edited volume presenting theory-driven, empirically based, developmentally oriented prevention." (Michael C. Roberts, PhD, Professor of Psychology, The University of Alabama)*

The National Mental Health Association: Eighty Years of Involvement in the Field of Prevention, edited by Robert E. Hess, PhD, and Jean DeLeon, PhD* (Vol. 6, No. 2, 1989). *"As a family life educator interested in both the history of the field, current efforts, and especially the evaluation of programs, I find this book quite interesting. I enjoyed reviewing it and believe that I will return to it many times. It is also a book I will recommend to students." (Family Relations)*

A Guide to Conducting Prevention Research in the Community: First Steps, by James G. Kelly, PhD, Nancy Dassoff, PhD, Ira Levin, PhD, Janice Schreckengost, MA, AB, Stephen P. Stelzner, PhD, and B. Eileen Altman, PhD* (Vol. 6, No. 1, 1989). *"An invaluable compendium for the prevention practitioner, as well as the researcher, laying out the essentials for developing effective prevention programs in the community. . . . This is a book which should be in the prevention practitioner's library, to read, re-read, and ponder." (The Community Psychologist)*

Prevention: Toward a Multidisciplinary Approach, edited by Leonard A. Jason, PhD, Robert D. Felner, PhD, John N. Moritsugu, PhD, and Robert E. Hess, PhD* (Vol. 5, No. 2, 1987). *"Will not only be of intellectual value to the professional but also to students in courses aimed at presenting a refreshingly comprehensive picture of the conceptual and practical relationships between community and prevention." (Seymour B. Sarason, Associate Professor of Psychology, Yale University)*

Prevention and Health: Directions for Policy and Practice, edited by Alfred H. Katz, PhD, Jared A. Hermalin, PhD, and Robert E. Hess, PhD* (Vol. 5, No. 1, 1987). *Read about the most current efforts being undertaken to promote better health.*

The Ecology of Prevention: Illustrating Mental Health Consultation, edited by James G. Kelly, PhD, and Robert E. Hess, PhD* (Vol. 4, No. 3/4, 1987). *"Will provide the consultant with a very useful framework and the student with an appreciation for the time and commitment necessary to bring about lasting changes of a preventive nature." (The Community Psychologist)*

Beyond the Individual: Environmental Approaches and Prevention, edited by Abraham Wandersman, PhD, and Robert E. Hess, PhD* (Vol. 4, No. 1/2, 1985). *"This excellent book has immediate appeal for those involved with environmental psychology . . . likely to be of great interest to those working in the areas of community psychology, planning, and design." (Australian Journal of Psychology)*

Prevention: The Michigan Experience, edited by Betty Tableman, MPA, and Robert E. Hess, PhD* (Vol. 3, No. 4, 1985). *An in-depth look at one state's outstanding prevention programs.*

Studies in Empowerment: Steps Toward Understanding and Action, edited by Julian Rappaport, Carolyn Swift, and Robert E. Hess, PhD* (Vol. 3, No. 2/3, 1984). *"Provides diverse applications of the empowerment model to the promotion of mental health and the prevention of mental illness." (Prevention Forum Newsline)*

Aging and Prevention: New Approaches for Preventing Health and Mental Health Problems in Older Adults, edited by Sharon P. Simson, Laura Wilson, Jared Hermalin, PhD, and Robert E. Hess, PhD* (Vol. 3, No. 1, 1983). *"Highly recommended for professionals and laymen interested in modern viewpoints and techniques for avoiding many physical and mental health problems of the elderly. Written by highly qualified contributors with extensive experience in their respective fields." (The Clinical Gerontologist)*

Strategies for Needs Assessment in Prevention, edited by Alex Zautra, Kenneth Bachrach, and Robert E. Hess, PhD* (Vol. 2, No. 4, 1983). *"An excellent survey on applied techniques for doing needs assessments. . . . It should be on the shelf of anyone involved in prevention." (Journal of Pediatric Psychology)*

Innovations in Prevention, edited by Robert E. Hess, PhD, and Jared Hermalin, PhD* (Vol. 2, No. 3, 1983). *An exciting book that provides invaluable insights on effective prevention programs.*

Rx Television: Enhancing the Preventive Impact of TV, edited by Joyce Sprafkin, Carolyn Swift, PhD, and Robert E. Hess, PhD* (Vol. 2, No. 1/2, 1983). *"The successful interventions reported in this volume make interesting reading on two grounds. First, they show quite clearly how powerful television can be in molding children. Second, they illustrate how this power can be used for good ends." (Contemporary Psychology)*

Early Intervention Programs for Infants, edited by Howard A. Moss, MD, Robert E. Hess, PhD, and Carolyn Swift, PhD* (Vol. 1, No. 4, 1982). *"A useful resource book for those child psychiatrists, paediatricians, and psychologists interested in early intervention and prevention." (The Royal College of Psychiatrists)*

Helping People to Help Themselves: Self-Help and Prevention, edited by Leonard D. Borman, PhD, Leslie E. Borck, PhD, Robert E. Hess, PhD, and Frank L. Pasquale* (Vol. 1, No. 3, 1982). *"A timely volume . . . a mine of information for interested clinicians, and should stimulate those wishing to do systematic research in the self-help area." (The Journal of Nervous and Mental Disease)*

Evaluation and Prevention in Human Services, edited by Jared Hermalin, PhD, and Jonathan A. Morell, PhD* (Vol. 1, No. 1/2, 1982). *Features methods and problems related to the evaluation of prevention programs.*

Index

Abortion, forced, 26,32-33
Abuse, use of term, 57
Addiction Severity Index, 71
Adolescents
African-American boys, 5-19
control over one's body, 31-33
exposure to violence, 2,6,7-8,9,10, 13,26,40
girls in guerrilla forces, 26-36
sexual abuse of, 22,23-24,26,27, 32-33,35-36
sexual development of, 31-33
Adult romantic attachment
measure of, 54
sexual abuse and, 62
Africa, child soldiers in, 23,25-26
African-American youth, risk and
resiliency of, 5-19
Aftercare, 70,77
Age
spirituality and, 44,45
stressful life experiences and, 44,45
trauma symptoms and, 44,45
Aggression
assessment of, 11
and exposure to violence, 8,13
self-esteem and, 13
social support and, 7,8
Aggressive Behavior Scale, 11
Anxiety
assessment of, 11,55,73-74
and exposure to violence, 8
predictors of, 75
self-esteem and, 13
sexual abuse and, 61,62
Armed Revolutionary Forces of
Colombia (FARC), 21-23,26
Attachment, as foundation of
personality, 83-84

Attachment styles, 3-4
early studies of, 84
and history of abuse, 59, 61
measurement of, 85-90
of trauma therapists, 81-92
Avoidance, measurement of, 84,86-90

Beck Anxiety Inventory, 55
Beck Depression Inventory, 54-55
Bosnia, child soldiers in, 23,25

Children
attachment patterns in, 83-84
choices open to, 36
domestic violence in homes of, 27
in domestic violence shelters, 67, 69,72
human rights of, 22
physical abuse of, 28,29
of poverty, 22,27,29
sexual abuse (CSA) of see Sexual
abuse
war and, 21-24,26,35-36
Children's Coping Strategies
Checklist, 11-12
Children's Exposure to Violence
Scale, 10
Clinical elevations, abuse and, 60,61
Cognitive Distortion Scales, 53
Colombia
drug production in, 24
guerrilla in, 21-38
humanitarian emergency in, 24
patriarchy in, 28-30
rehabilitation in, 35-36
war in, 24-26,36
women's rights in, 24

exposure to, 2,6,7-8,9,10,13,26,40
intervention strategies and, 9,16
perception of, 14
sexual, 23-24,26,50
Virginity, proof of, 32

War
combat exposure in, 33-35
dissociation mechanisms in, 34-35
effects on children of, 21-24,26,
35-36
gender-distinct effects in, 23-24
military tasks in, 31
survival strategies in, 24-25
and trauma experience, 25-26
West Bank and Occupied Territories,
child soldiers in, 23
Women
in abusive relationships, 68-71
and division of labor, 23,30-31

domestic violence shelters for,
67-80
human rights of, 24
of poverty, 25
in recovery programs, 3
sexual abuse reported by, 49-65
sexual exploitation of, 23-24
sexual violence against, 23-24,26,
50,68-71
survival strategies of, 24-25
therapists, 3,81-92
victimization of, 68-71
war and, 23-24
Wyatt Sexual History Questionnaire,
53,56-57

Young Schema Questionnaire, 53-54
Youth Self-Report (YSR), 11